THE NEW CARB CYCLING SYSTEM

Discover the Ultimate 3 Meal Plans Method for Effective Weight Loss
Through Alternating Carbohydrates

Cicely Vanwinkle

1

TABLE OF CONTENTS

INTRODUCTION

Welcome to the gateway of your transformation journey where the harmonious balance of knowledge and action fosters profound changes. With "The New Carb Cycling System," you are not just reading another diet book; you are stepping into a tested method intertwined with the science of nutrition and the art of personal commitment. This book is our rendezvous point—a starting line from where you'll embark on a path carved by clarity, scientific wisdom, and personal anecdotes that illustrate the reachable reality of effective weight management.

Carb cycling, as you will discover, is not merely an eating pattern, but a dynamic way to enhance your body's metabolic responses. It's both a foundation and a flexible plan tailored to work with the personal rhythm of your life—encompassing busy work schedules, family meals, and even those unavoidable social gatherings. It's designed with you in mind, acknowledging that life doesn't stop while you're trying to improve your health.

Throughout these pages, we will debunk the myths that have perhaps cluttered your path to wellness before. We'll explore how alternating carbohydrate intake not only aids in achieving and maintaining your ideal weight but also in enhancing your energy levels and overall health. The essence of carb cycling lies in its adaptability to your individual life—as dynamic and changing as it may be.

Imagine this book as a conversation between friends, one of whom just happens to be armed with expertise in nutrition and a passion for wellness. Our dialogue will walk you through the foundational science behind the strategy, easing into practical and actionable steps that you can integrate seamlessly into your day-to-day life.

By the time you turn the final page, "The New Carb Cycling System" will have hopefully shifted from being a book to your trusty companion in the journey towards sustainable health. Let's begin this adventure together, equipped with knowledge and motivated by the clear, attainable goals we will set together.

WELCOME

Welcome to a journey that transcends the ordinary path of dieting to embrace a lifestyle of informed, dynamic nutrition management. If you've ever felt lost in the sea of conflicting dietary advice or struggled to keep up with the latest fitness trends, this book promises a different narrative, one that respects the nuances of your individual lifestyle while guiding you towards sustainable weight loss and improved health.

Carb cycling is not a magic bullet; it is a well-researched, flexible strategy that allows you to align your carbohydrate intake with your body's needs, making weight loss more manageable and less restrictive. The true beauty of carb cycling lies in its adaptability—it bends to the curve of your life's rhythms, accommodating periods of activity and rest, celebration and everyday routine.

At its core, carb cycling rotates between high-carb days and low-carb days. This method helps in optimizing your body's metabolic processes and managing energy levels efficiently. On high-carb days, you fuel your body for more strenuous activities, capitalizing on the energy that carbohydrates provide. On low-carb days, you encourage your body to tap into fat stores for fuel, aiding in effective weight management and body composition changes.

This nuanced approach to eating is particularly advantageous for those who have experienced the frustrating plateau effect inherent in so many other dietary plans. By fluctuating carbohydrate intake, your body remains off-balance in a controlled, strategic way that can prevent these plateaus, keeping your metabolic rate more responsive and engaged.

As we delve into the mechanisms behind this system, it's important to anchor our discussion in the reality of day-to-day challenges. Integrating carb cycling into your life doesn't require perfection. Instead, it's about making more informed choices that align with your body's needs. Whether you are eating out with friends, spending time with family, or traveling, this system provides guidelines that can adapt to various social settings and personal preferences.

Carb cycling also honors the multifaceted nature of food—as nourishment, as pleasure, as culture, and as comfort. It's not just about counting carbs; it's about understanding how different foods can fuel different kinds of activities and moods, and how you can leverage this understanding to improve your health without giving up the joy of eating.

Let me share a story of one of the early adopters of this method from our community. Emily, a 35-year-old mother of two, struggled with yo-yo dieting for years, each new diet promising a lot but delivering little in the way of sustainable change. Carb cycling, however, offered her not just a diet plan but a new perspective on food. She learned how her body responded to different types of food and started enjoying cooking different meals designed for high-carb and low-carb days. Through carb cycling, Emily didn't just lose weight—she gained an empowering understanding of her nutritional needs and a way to fulfill them without feeling deprived or exhausted.

As we progress through the book, each chapter will build on the last, creating a comprehensive guide that covers everything from understanding the basic principles of carb cycling to gradually implementing and mastering it. Each section is designed to provide practical advice that you can start using immediately, supplemented by insights into the science behind why these strategies work.

This is not just about changing how you eat; it's about changing how you think about eating and about your body. It's about equipping you with knowledge and tools that empower you to make decisions that feel good and are good for you.

Carb cycling acknowledges that life is unpredictable and eating should be enjoyable. Throughout this guide, I will share tips on how you can stay flexible and maintain your commitment even when life gets chaotic. We'll explore how to handle dining out, what to do when you're traveling, and how to manage special occasions—from birthdays to holidays—without veering off track.

The route to wellness through carb cycling is as much about understanding your physiological responses as it is about recognizing and respecting your emotional and psychological needs related to food and eating. This book aims to support your journey on all these levels, ensuring that your path towards health is as fulfilling and rewarding as it is effective.

By embracing carb cycling as a lifestyle, rather than a strict diet, you open up a new way of living where each meal is an opportunity to support your body's health, your mind's happiness, and your spirit's zest for life. Let us begin this transformative journey together, with open minds and adventurous hearts. Welcome to the world of informed, enjoyable, and sustainable eating.

THE SCIENCE BEHIND CARB CYCLING

Carbohydrates have often been painted as villains in the narrative of nutrition and weight loss. But what if I told you that carbs, when understood and utilized correctly, could be your most powerful ally in achieving a sculpted physique and vibrant health? This premise is not born from a whimsical desire to rebel against low-carb dogmas, but from solid scientific research. The practice of carb cycling leverages the body's natural response to carbohydrates, juggling high-carb and low-carb days to ignite your metabolism and catalyze fat loss without sacrificing muscle mass or energy levels.

Understanding how carb cycling works at a scientific level can be both enlightening and empowering. Our bodies are wonderfully complex systems capable of remarkable adaptability, and carb cycling speaks to this very flexibility. On high-carb days, your body's insulin response is activated. Insulin, a hormone produced by the pancreas, facilitates the transport of glucose into the cells where it is utilized for energy. It's during these high-carb phases that your body replenishes glycogen stores, which fuels muscular activity and supports overall energy levels.

Low-carb days, in contrast, encourage your body to turn to stored fat for fuel. This process, known as ketosis, happens when the intake of carbohydrates is limited enough that the body begins to break down fat for energy, resulting in fat loss. Meanwhile, the alternation between low and high-carb days aims to prevent the metabolic slowdown associated with continuous calorie restriction.

However, the effectiveness of carbohydrate cycling transcends the biochemical narrative of hormones and metabolism. It also harmonizes with our psychological needs for variety and satisfaction in our diet, which can significantly boost compliance and long-term success. This duality of satisfaction—meeting both physiological needs and psychological desires—is what makes carb cycling a uniquely sustainable approach to fitness and health.

Consider the challenges faced by 'Jenny', a composite of many who have walked through the doors of diet despair. She had tried strict, low-carb diets before; each time, initial success was wiped away by fatigue, irritability, and a creeping sense of deprivation which culminated in binge eating. Carb cycling's approach, with its intrinsic balance and rhythm, presented a different narrative to her, one where no food group was the enemy and her energy levels could remain buoyant.

Jenny's experience mirrors the findings of clinical studies where participants exhibited improved body composition, better-controlled insulin and glucose levels, and enhanced physical performance when following a carb cycling protocol as compared to traditional dieting. For instance, a research study highlighted that athletes who practiced carb cycling were able to maintain more muscle mass and sustain a higher metabolism compared to their peers on low-carb diets.

It's important to note that while carb cycling has its roots in bodybuilding and elite athletics, its principles are universally applicable. The fundamental science—manipulating carb intake to manipulate metabolic responses—can be adapted by anyone. Whether you're an office worker, a busy parent, or a fitness enthusiast, the ability to use carbs strategically can help you reach your weight loss goals while still enjoying the nutritional benefits of whole grains, fruits, and vegetables on high-carb days.

Moreover, the strategic increase in carbohydrate intake on specific days or periods serves more than just replenishing glycogen stores; it also boosts leptin, the satiety hormone, which can help regulate appetite and prevent overeating. This is why carb cycling can be particularly beneficial for those who have reached a plateau in their weight loss journey—the strategic spikes in carb intake can help reset hormonal balance and jump-start metabolic rates.

In embracing carb cycling, we're not just subscribing to a diet but aligning ourselves with a broader understanding of how our bodies function. It's about respecting the natural rhythms of our metabolism and using science to turn the tables on the typical feast-or-famine scenario posed by many diets. By cycling our carb intake, we provide our bodies with what they need, when they need it, supporting an optimal balance of fat loss, muscle maintenance, and energy levels.

As we delve deeper into the following chapters, the mechanisms of carb cycling will be unpacked with more granularity. We'll explore how you can tailor this approach to fit your individual lifestyle and goals, backed by actionable advice and driven by scientific integrity. Remember, the essence of this journey is grounded in a compassionate understanding of human biology and the desire for a realistic, flexible approach to eating—one that champions variety, balance, and sustained satisfaction in your dieting endeavors.

HOW TO USE THIS BOOK

Imagine this book as a toolkit designed specifically with your needs in mind—versatile, detailed, and informative, yet flexible enough to accommodate your unique lifestyle. "The New Carb Cycling System" is as much a guide to understanding the relationship between your diet and your body as it is a compass to steering you towards your optimal health and fitness goals.

From the very beginning, it's crucial to approach this book not just as a reader, but as an engaged participant in your health journey. The chapters are laid out to subtly guide you through the preliminary concepts and into the more intricate strategies of carb cycling, ensuring that regardless of your previous experiences with diets or health regimes, you are well-prepared to apply these principles effectively.

Start with a solid foundation by thoroughly understanding the concepts explained in the first few chapters. Here, you'll grasp the 'whys' and 'hows' of carb cycling, which will support your journey. Knowing the science behind the process and the reasons for each step will not only motivate you but also help you make informed decisions when faced with dietary choices.

Onward from the foundational knowledge, we transition to practical application in later chapters. This section is the heart of the book, designed for you to start applying the concepts to your daily life.

Each chapter builds on the previous ones, so while it's tempting to jump straight to the meal plans and recipes, understanding the underlying principles listed earlier will enhance your ability to use these tools effectively.

Each chapter concludes with actionable steps that you can begin to integrate immediately into your routine. These activities range from tracking your current eating habits, structuring your meal preparations, to gradually introducing changes to your diet. These steps are designed to be actionable and manageable, making the transition to a carb cycling diet as smooth as possible.

As you navigate through the book, use the chapters as checkpoints, pausing at each to assess your understanding and comfort level with the information. This is not a race to the finish line but a journey towards better health and understanding of your body. If at any point you feel overwhelmed, take a moment to revisit the earlier concepts or reach out to a community of fellow readers to share tips, questions, and successes.

Moreover, keep a journal as you go through this process. Documenting your meals, how you feel physically and emotionally, and any changes you notice in your body can provide invaluable feedback. This personal record is not just a log but a mirror reflecting back your progress, struggles, and insights—it's a critical tool that complements the scientific information in this book.

For those particularly committed to digging deeper, references and further reading suggestions are included to enrich your understanding of carb cycling. These resources are an excellent way to expand your knowledge and provide a broader context to what is shared in the book.

On practical days when meal prep seems like a chore or temptation looms, remind yourself of the stories and case studies shared within these pages. Real-life examples serve as motivational reminders that your goals are achievable, and that many before you have successfully navigated this journey.

Lastly, this book is designed to be revisited as your relationship with food and understanding of your body evolves. Your first read-through might surface questions and highlight areas needing more focus, which is entirely expected. As you grow more accustomed to carb cycling, you'll find that different sections of the book resonate differently, providing new insights each time.

By the end of this book, you'll not only have a thorough understanding of carb cycling but possess a personalized approach to integrating these practices into your life effectively. This journey is about transforming your health, energizing your body, and elevating your understanding of nutrition's role in overall wellness. So, take a deep breath, turn the page, and let's begin this transformative exploration together.

CHAPTER 1: UNDERSTANDING CARB CYCLING

As we embark on a journey through the intriguing world of carb cycling, it's essential to first establish a solid understanding of what carb cycling truly is and how it can transform your approach to dieting and weight management. Imagine a method that flexibly adapts to your lifestyle, alleviating the monotony of conventional diets while boosting your metabolic health and fostering weight loss. This is the heart of carb cycling—a powerful strategy tailored for those who seek sustainable weight loss without sacrificing their love for food.

Carb cycling is not just another diet trend; it's a scientifically grounded approach that alternates between high-carb and low-carb days. This rhythmic variation in carbohydrate intake works harmoniously with your body's natural energy needs, maximizing fat loss and muscle preservation. On days when you're more active, higher carb intake fuels your strenuous activities, whereas low-carb days help you tap into stored fat for energy, thereby enhancing your weight loss effort.

This chapter will guide you through the core principles of carb cycling, debunk the myths that often cloud its true benefits, and provide a clearer picture of why alternating carbohydrate intake could be the key to unlocking a healthier, more energized you. As we delve deeper, we'll explore how this method not only supports weight loss but also strengthens your body's metabolic flexibility—enabling you to enjoy a broader range of foods and, ultimately, lead a more balanced life.

Understanding the principles behind carb cycling will empower you to tailor this method to your individual needs, making it a perfect fit for your busy schedule and diverse dietary preferences. It's about creating harmony between your body's physiological needs and your personal life commitments—an approach that doesn't just change how you eat, but enhances how you live.

So, let's set aside any preconceived notions about dieting and explore how the adaptable, effective strategy of carb cycling can be seamlessly integrated into your lifestyle, helping you achieve and maintain your weight loss goals with vitality and zest. Join me in discovering how to turn the science of carb cycling into a practical, enjoyable part of your daily routine.

1. THE BASICS OF CARB CYCLING

Imagine if you could manipulate your diet to fit not only your nutritional needs but your daily life's rhythm as well—syncing your eating habits with your body's natural energy demands. This is precisely where the concept of carb cycling shines, a method that allows for flexibility and structure, providing an essential balance in today's fast-paced world.

Carb cycling is a dietary approach where you alternate carbohydrate intake on a daily, weekly, or monthly basis. It is often used to lose weight, maintain physical performance while dieting, or overcome a weight loss plateau. At its core, carb cycling manipulates your body's metabolism and can be tailored to support different fitness goals, whether it be fat loss, muscle gain, or a combination of both.

On a high-carb day, when your body receives more carbohydrates than usual, it boosts your insulin levels and energy, making it ideal for fueling intensive physical activities.

On the contrary, low-carb days may make your body more apt to turn fat into energy, promoting fat loss. This shift can help you manage or lose weight while still enjoying the benefits of carbohydrates paradoxically.

Benefits of Carb Cycling

The beauty of carb cycling lies in its versatility and the array of benefits it offers. For starters, it aligns with natural hormonal fluctuations, optimizing when your body utilizes carbs for energy or fat storage. One of the most prominent benefits of this method is avoiding the plateau effect commonly associated with more traditional diets, where metabolic rates dip due to constant calorie or macronutrient intake.

Moreover, carb cycling allows for higher carbohydrate days, which can increase glycogen stores and boost performance in the gym. This is particularly beneficial for those who engage in high-intensity workouts as it provides the necessary energy without the constant feeling of deprivation associated with typical diets.

For those who worry about the mental fog and fatigue often associated with low-carb diets, carb cycling offers a respite. High-carb days help replenish glycogen stores, enhancing mood and cognitive function. Furthermore, the flexibility of the carb cycling plan helps maintain a person's motivation and adherence to their diet because it is less restrictive overall, making it a sustainable long-term approach to nutrition.

Myths and Misconceptions

Despite its benefits, there are several myths surrounding carb cycling that might deter people from considering this effective dietary strategy. One common myth is that carb cycling is overly complex and strict. On the contrary, while it does require some initial planning, once you are accustomed to the cyclical pattern, it becomes just as easy to follow as any diet plan.

Another popular misconception is that carb cycling is only for athletes or individuals with a significant amount of weight to lose. This is not the case. Carb cycling can be beneficial for anyone looking to improve their body composition, energy levels, and overall health. It is adaptable to all fitness levels and goals and can be modified for those who are just starting their fitness journey or those who need a new strategy after hitting a plateau.

There is also a myth that suggests carb cycling negatively impacts metabolism because of intermittent low-carb intake. However, the strategic, cyclical increase in carbs ensures that your metabolism does not slow down. By alternating, you keep your body guessing, which can maintain or even enhance your metabolic rate over time.

Moving from Theory to Practice

Understanding the basics of carb cycling paves the way for implementing it effectively in your own life. Whether your goal is to lose weight, gain muscle, or break through a frustrating plateau, carb cycling can be an invaluable tool. The key to success lies in customizing your carb intake days to align with your activity levels and personal goals while maintaining a balanced intake of proteins and fats to support overall health.

The next step is practical application: setting realistic, achievable goals based on your lifestyle and nutritional needs.

By integrating high and low-carb days, you can guide your body towards better performance and optimal energy usage throughout your weight management journey. As you learn to listen to your body's signals and adjust your intake accordingly, you'll find more than just success in carb cycling—you'll discover a flexible approach to eating that can be maintained long term for sustained health and vitality.

In summary, carb cycling is not only about shedding pounds or muscle building; it's about creating a harmonious relationship with food that respects your body's natural rhythms and needs. As we continue our journey in the following chapters, we will delve into how to effectively devise a carb cycling plan that fits seamlessly into your life, ensuring you reap all the potential benefits this strategy has to offer.

2. How Carb Cycling Works

Understanding the detailed mechanics of carb cycling can empower you to utilize its fullest potential in aligning with your lifestyle and your body's natural processes. Delving into how high-carb and low-carb days function and the critical role of proteins and fats will not only optimize your results but also enhance your overall well-being and diet satisfaction.

How High-Carb Days Benefit You

In the dance of carb cycling, high-carb days are like the crescendos in a symphony, providing energy and vitality. These days are strategically aligned with your most intense physical activities, such as heavy lifting or long-duration cardio, when your body demands more fuel. On high-carb days, your body's insulin sensitivity is at its peak. Consuming more carbohydrates on these days ensures that glucose is efficiently stored in the muscles and liver as glycogen rather than being converted to fat. This is not merely about boosting your energy for workouts; it's about maximizing recovery, promoting muscle growth, and enhancing your body's ability to repair itself after strenuous activity.

When you ingest carbohydrates, they are broken down into sugars that enter your bloodstream. Insulin then shuttles these sugars into cells, primarily muscle cells, to be used as energy or stored for future use. This process helps maintain blood sugar levels within a healthy range and ensures your muscles have the energy they are likely to require for increased activity. As a result, on high-carb days, not only are your physical vigor and stamina enhanced, but your muscle recovery and growth are also supported more effectively.

The Strategic Reduction on Low-Carb Days

After the high comes the calm—the low-carb days. These days support your body's fat-burning processes. With reduced carbohydrate intake, your body is prompted to turn to stored fat for energy. This switch is crucial for effective weight management and body composition improvements. By reducing your carb intake, insulin levels lower, which facilitates fat breakdown and usage. These days should ideally be scheduled on your less active days, where intense bursts of energy are not required but maintaining a steady, functional energy level is still crucial.

On low-carb days, your body enhances its capability to metabolize fat for fuel, a metabolic flexibility that can lead to improved overall health and energy efficiency. The practice of moderating carb intake intermittently also aids your body in maintaining insulin sensitivity, which is crucial for long-term metabolic health and preventing conditions like diabetes.

Balancing the Scale with Proteins and Fats

While carbohydrates are the main actors changing scenes in carb cycling, proteins and fats provide the continuous support that keeps the show running smoothly. Proteins are vital for muscle repair and growth, especially important given the variable carb intake's effect on muscle synthesis. On both high-carb and low-carb days, maintaining a steady, adequate protein intake is crucial. Proteins help stabilize blood sugar levels, reduce hunger by increasing satiety, and prevent muscle loss, especially on low-carb days when your body might otherwise seek to use muscle tissue for energy.

Fats, often unjustly vilified, are actually critical to your body's long-term energy needs, hormone function, and absorption of fat-soluble vitamins. On low-carb days, fats become particularly important. They provide a consistent energy source that complements the body's increased reliance on fat for energy. Healthy fats from sources like avocados, nuts, seeds, and fish support cellular function and health, contributing to inflammatory responses and maintaining brain health.

In the grand schema of carb cycling, understanding how to implement high-carb and low-carb days alongside a continuous intake of proteins and fats requires knowing more than just your schedule. It involves recognizing your body's signals—how it responds to varying activity levels and dietary changes. This harmony between active and restful days, fueled appropriately by carbs, supported unwaveringly by proteins and fats, creates a rhythm to your eating pattern that fosters not only effective weight management but a holistic well-being.

The interplay of macronutrients in carb cycling reveals a dynamic and sophisticated approach to eating. It's more than altering your carb consumption; it's about creating a flexible, responsive feeding strategy that supports your energy needs, fitness goals, and overall health. As you move forward, integrating high-carb and low-carb days will become as natural as listening to your body's cues for rest and activity—and as gratifying as meeting those needs efficiently. This foundational knowledge not only sets the stage for a deeper dive into personalized meal planning but also positions you to adjust and succeed in your carb cycling journey with confidence.

3. SETTING REALISTIC GOALS

Embarking on a journey of transformation through carb cycling begins with the cornerstone of all great endeavors: setting realistic goals. This step, integral yet often overlooked, requires us to engage in soul-searching and precise strategizing. What do you hope to achieve? Whether it's shedding those stubborn last few pounds, enhancing athletic performance, or simply feeling more energized, your goals will direct every aspect of your carb cycling plan.

Defining Your Goals

Consider, for a moment, your lifestyle, responsibilities, and limitations all shaped by your unique narrative. Within this context, setting goals for carb cycling should be a reflection of what is simultaneously challenging and achievable. Goals should stretch your abilities but remain firmly rooted in the realistic. They are not just about the destination but are carved into meaningful steps that map out your journey.

Think in terms of specific, measurable, achievable, relevant, and time-bound (SMART) objectives. For instance, rather than a vague goal like 'lose weight,' specify 'lose 10 pounds in 12 weeks using the carb cycling method.' This clear, targeted goal not only states what you wish to accomplish but also incorporates a method and a timeframe, making it easier to monitor and adjust as you progress.

Tracking Progress

As you implement carb cycling, it's crucial to monitor your progress objectively. This isn't solely about stepping onto a scale; it's about understanding how different aspects of your life are responding to your new eating pattern. Remember, your relationship with food and your body is deeply personal and multifaceted. Hence, tracking shouldn't just be about numbers. How do you feel? Are your energy levels higher? Are you starting to see improvements in your physical strength or endurance? Answers to these questions are qualitative but hugely significant markers of progress.

Today, we have a broad range of tools at our disposal for tracking—from apps that log your daily carb intake to more traditional methods like food diaries and workout logs. These tools can help provide insights into how well your body is adapting to carb cycling and where adjustments might be needed. Furthermore, periodic photos, body measurements, and muscle mass analysis can offer a broader picture of the changes occurring in your body, beyond the basic metric of weight.

Adjusting Your Plan

Adaptability is crucial in every life plan, and carb cycling is no exception. Sometimes, the feedback from your body or your tracking tool of choice will suggest that your initial goals are too ambitious or too mild. Or perhaps life's unforeseen hurdles, like an illness or heightened work stress, may interfere with your progress. These are not signs of failure but opportunities to reassess and recalibrate your approach.

Adjusting your carb cycling plan requires an honest evaluation of what is working and what isn't. It might mean altering your high-carb and low-carb days, adjusting caloric intake, or changing the types of carbohydrates consumed. For many, it also involves reassessing their relationship with food and body image, ensuring that psychological well-being is maintained alongside physical health.

Moreover, support during these adjustments is invaluable. Whether it's a nutritionist, a personal trainer, or a community of fellow carb cyclers, having a robust support system can provide motivation, insights, and encouragement. These resources can be pivotal in helping you navigate the challenges of adjusting your plan and can empower you to make informed, effective changes.

Through this cyclical process of setting goals, tracking progress, and making necessary adjustments, you engage in an ongoing dialogue with your body and lifestyle. This cycle is not just about transformation but about integration—integrating a new way of eating into your life in a way that feels as natural and sustaining as possible.

In essence, defining realistic goals, keeping accurate tabs on your progress, and being willing to make adjustments are not just steps in managing your carb cycling plan—they are affirmations of your commitment to your health and well-being. As you move through this process, each small milestone brings you closer not only to your physical goals but also to a deeper understanding of your body's needs and rhythms. As challenging as it might be, the journey through carb cycling is as rewarding as reaching your final destination, equipped with insights and habits that will serve you well beyond your immediate goals.

CHAPTER 2: NUTRITIONAL FOUNDATIONS

Embarking on your journey through the world of carb cycling, understanding the pillars of nutrition is paramount. As we delve into the fundamentals, envision these elements as the frame of a house, holding everything together and upholding the structure that supports your weight loss and wellness goals. This chapter, "Nutritional Foundations," sets the stage to unpack the complexities of macronutrients, hydration, and how they interplay with your carb cycling efforts. Consider the profound relationship you have with food—it's not only fuel but a source of joy, a part of celebrations, and sometimes, a balm for the soul. The nutrients you consume craft the pages of your body's story, influencing energy levels, metabolic functions, and even mood. Our focus on macronutrients—carbohydrates, proteins, and fats—extends beyond mere definitions. It explores their pivotal roles and how they collaborate to bolster your health.

Carbohydrates often wear the villain's cape in diet narratives, but here, we reframe them as the versatile and vital resources they are, especially in a well-orchestrated carb cycling plan. Proteins, renowned for their muscle-building prowess, also have a cameo in various other crucial roles, from healing to hormonal balance. Fats, once unjustly exiled from healthy diets, return as essential heroes in hormone production and nutrient absorption.

Transitioning to micronutrients, think of these as the fine tools in your wellness toolbox—small but mighty. They ensure the smooth operation of bodily functions and fortify your defenses. Hydration, too, plays a non-negotiable role, akin to the lifeblood of your cells, facilitating every process in your body.

This chapter aims not just to educate but to empower you with knowledge that can be seamlessly woven into the fabric of your daily life. As we peel back the layers of nutrient interactions and their impacts, you'll discover how to balance your plate with an artist's touch—combining colors, textures, and nutrients to fuel both body and spirit on your carb cycling journey. Together, we'll build a foundation robust and resilient enough to support not just a diet, but a thriving, vibrant lifestyle.

1. MACRONUTRIENTS 101

When navigating the landscape of nutrition, especially within the framework of carb cycling, the broad categories of macronutrients—carbohydrates, proteins, and fats—serve as your compasses. These are not just abstract components listed on the back of food packages but vital elements that fuel your everyday activities and, importantly, your transformative journey on a carb cycling diet.

Understanding Carbohydrates: The Fuel for Your Fires

Carbohydrates often bear much controversy; demonized by some diets, hailed by others, their true significance is found in balance and quality. Carbs are your body's preferred energy source, broken down into glucose, the fuel that powers everything from rigorous workouts to your quietest breaths. They are not merely energy capsules; they are fibers and starches, each type playing distinct roles.

The fiber in carbohydrates, particularly from whole sources like fruits, vegetables, and whole grains, is pivotal. While it doesn't convert to glucose, fiber aids digestion, helps regulate blood sugar levels, and even prolongs feelings of fullness, all of which are crucial when attempting to manage weight and improve health. Fiber's role in our diet extends to influencing gut health, which recent science links to everything from immune function to mood regulation.

On carb cycling, high-carb days aren't about indulgence but strategic fueling. Your high-carb intake days should coincide with higher intensity workout days. On these days, whole grains, fruits, and vegetables aren't merely components of a meal but tools that refill glycogen stores, enhance recovery, and prepare the body for subsequent exertions.

The Importance of Proteins: More Than Muscle

Proteins break down into amino acids, the building blocks of almost every cellular process in the body. This macronutrient's fame comes from its role in building and repairing muscles, but its job description spans far broader. Proteins are instrumental in forming hormones, enzymes, and other critical biochemical components.

One of the essential features of protein, particularly within the carb cycling framework, is its satiating power, which can help curb the hunger and potential overeating on lower carbohydrate days. For instance, integrating lean meats, legumes, or dairy into meals provides a sustained energy release, which helps maintain blood sugar levels and staves off cravings.

For those involved in weight training or heavy physical activities, protein's importance magnifies as it helps repair and build new muscle tissue stressed during exercise. However, the magic of protein is in its thermogenic effect—it actually requires more energy to metabolize compared to carbs and fats, effectively increasing caloric burn while digesting.

Healthy Fats and Their Role: The Misunderstood Macronutrient

Fats have long been vilified; however, they are essential not only for health but as a cornerstone of sustained weight loss and energy management in carb cycling. Fats are dense forms of energy, crucial for the absorption of fat-soluble vitamins like A, D, E, and K. They are integral to building cell membranes and protective myelin sheaths around your nerves.

Moreover, fats contribute to hormone synthesis and regulation, including hormones like estrogen and testosterone, which are crucial for muscle growth and overall health. In the context of carb cycling, fats are particularly useful on low-carb days. They provide a steadier, more prolonged energy source, keeping you satiated longer, which can help manage the lower energy intake from reduced carbohydrates.

Choosing the right types of fats is paramount. Focus on unsaturated fats found in olive oil, avocados, and nuts, and be wary of trans fats, which can increase the risk of heart disease. Omega-3 fatty acids, found in fatty fish, flaxseeds, and walnuts, are particularly beneficial for their anti-inflammatory properties, which can support recovery and overall health.

In exploring the nuanced roles of macronutrients, it's evident that each plays a multifaceted role in not just maintaining health but enhancing it. As you apply carb cycling to your life, understanding these roles allows you to make informed choices about what to eat and when, aligning your diet with your body's needs across differing days of activity and rest.

The symphony of macronutrients in your diet must be fine-tuned to echo the demands of your lifestyle, workouts, and personal goals. On days packed with physical challenges, carbohydrates scale up to meet your dynamic needs, while recovery days highlight proteins and fats, allowing the body to rebuild and reshape. Through the intelligent application of these macronutrient principles, you're not just eating; you're engineering a diet that dynamically supports your evolving lifestyle and ambitions.

2. MICRONUTRIENTS AND HYDRATION

As we waltz further into the nuances of nutrition essential for optimizing the carb cycling method, it's paramount to turn our focus towards the often-overlooked, yet crucially significant, cast of nutrients: micronutrients and the elemental component of life—water. Though micronutrients—including vitamins and minerals—do not supply energy themselves like macronutrients, they are indispensable conductors orchestrating a range of bodily symphonies from bone health to immune support.

Essential Vitamins and Minerals: Tiny Tools with Tremendous Tasks

Imagine your body as a complex machine, where various biochemical reactions take place every second. Here, vitamins and minerals are the indispensable tools that help drive these essential processes. They are the unsung heroes in processes such as bone formation, blood coagulation, and cellular energy production. Each vitamin and mineral has a unique role; for instance, Vitamin D is paramount not only for calcium absorption, essential for bone density and health, but also for its potential roles in mood regulation and immune function.

Minerals like iron play a critical part in oxygen transport throughout the body, crucial for energy and performance, particularly in a physically demanding lifestyle. Magnesium, another quiet achiever, supports over 300 biochemical reactions, including nerve and muscle function — essential for every carb cycling phase.

Yet, despite their necessity, our bodies cannot self-produce many essential vitamins and minerals in sufficient amounts. Thus, ensuring a diet diverse in fruits, vegetables, nuts, seeds, whole grains, and lean proteins becomes not just a choice for variety but a necessity for nutritional completeness.

The Role of Supplements: Helping Hand or Unneeded Crutch?

In a perfect world, our plates would always overflow with nutrient-dense foods, providing us with our full spectrum of vitamins and minerals. The reality, however, often diverges from this ideal. Busy schedules, food preferences, and other practical hurdles can lead to gaps in our nutrition. Here, supplements can step in as valuable allies.

However, the line between useful and excessive is thin. It's vital to approach supplements with a strategy—use them to supplement, not replace, a healthy diet. For those on carb cycling, certain days might have reduced intake of specific food groups, potentially calling for targeted supplementation. For instance, on low-carb days, one might not consume enough fruits, which might justify a Vitamin C supplement.

It's also wise to consult with a healthcare provider before starting any supplement routine, especially to avoid exceeding safe levels of nutrient intake and to ensure the chosen supplements do not interfere with other health conditions or medications.

Staying Hydrated: The Essence of Life

Water is perhaps the most understated nutrient in the diet. It plays a role not just in hydration but in practically every biological function, including digestion, nutrient transport, and temperature regulation. For those navigating the waves of carb cycling, staying adequately hydrated is non-negotiable. Water requirements can surge on high-carb days, as carbohydrates require water for storage.

Drinking sufficient water supports the kidneys in excreting metabolic wastes produced during increased metabolic activities on high-carb days. Furthermore, adequate hydration can aid in appetite control—a boon for those looking to lose weight. It's often easy to mistake thirst for hunger, so keeping a bottle of water handy could be one of the simplest yet most effective strategies in your nutrition toolkit.

Hydration isn't just about drinking eight glasses of water a day; it involves understanding and listening to your body's signals. The color of your urine is a practical hydration indicator: Pale, straw-colored urine typically indicates good hydration, while a darker color might suggest a need to drink more water.

In the grand diagram of your dietary strategy, envision micronutrients as the meticulous tweaks and adjustments in machinery, necessary for optimal performance and longevity. Supplements, when used wisely, act as the necessary patches when there are gaps. And water, akin to the oil in an engine, is essential for smooth and efficient operation.

Together, these components of your diet build a robust framework, ensuring that your body is not just functioning but thriving under the demands of carb cycling. By understanding and implementing these principles, you empower yourself with more than just knowledge—you equip your body to reach and sustain its utmost potential, paving the way for a healthier, more vibrant life.

3. BALANCING YOUR DIET

As we explore the nutritional building blocks essential for the efficacious implementation of a carb cycling regimen, a pivotal concept we must address is the balance of your diet. This involves more than just choosing the right types of food; it requires attention to portion control, the timing of your meals, and proficiency in reading nutrition labels.

These elements are the fine tuners of your nutritional orchestra, crucial for harmonizing your day-to-day diet with your body's requirements and goals.

Portion Control: Mastering the Scale of Consumption

Portion control is critical, particularly within a carb cycling framework, where the quantity of food varies based on daily carbohydrate intake levels. Not merely a method to prevent overeating, portion control is an art that helps manage energy intake and is a precursor to achieving and maintaining a healthy weight. It's about understanding how much your body needs at different times of the day, aligning with both low and high-carb days effectively.

Visual cues can be a beneficial guide. For example, a serving of protein like meat or fish should be about the size of your palm. This intuitive method helps to prevent overindulgence but also ensures that you ingest enough nutrients on lower intake days. For those new to portion control, using smaller plates for meals can psychologically feel satisfying, helping to enjoy a full plate of food without overeating. Another technique is to focus on high-volume, low-calorie foods like leafy greens or broth-based soups that fill you up without significantly affecting your caloric intake.

Timing Your Meals: The Rhythm of Eating

In carb cycling, not only is what you eat important but when you eat plays a substantial role as well. The timing of your meals can influence everything from metabolic rates to hormone levels. Structuring your meals to suit your daily activities helps in optimizing energy use and storage. On high-carb days, timing carbohydrate intake around workouts can maximize glycogen storage and recovery, while on low-carb days, focusing more on fats and proteins can provide sustained energy without spikes in blood sugar.

Many find success with a consistent eating schedule as it helps regulate the body's internal clock and can improve sleep, mood, and energy levels. Eating your last meal of the day at least a couple of hours before bedtime is also a practice that can enhance sleep quality while aiding in digestion and metabolism throughout the night.

Reading Nutrition Labels: Decoding Dietary Data

In an age where food comes packaged in all forms, understanding nutrition labels is more crucial than ever. These labels are your primary tool for making informed food choices that align with your dietary requirements on both high and low-carb days. Start by looking at the serving size and compare it with the amount you consume; this will guide you in understanding the total nutrients you intake from a particular food item.

Key components on the label like total fats, carbohydrates, dietary fibers, sugars, and proteins give insight into how well-suited a food is to your carb cycling plan. For instance, on low-carb days, foods higher in protein and fat are preferable, whereas high-carb days can accommodate more from the total carbohydrates section, particularly if these carbs are coming from whole sources like whole grains and not just sugars.

Moreover, paying attention to the micronutrient section can ensure you're not missing out on essential vitamins and minerals, especially during restrictive phases. Another critical element is the ingredient list, which should ideally be short and filled with recognizable items. It's a simple rule: the fewer the ingredients, the less processed the food, and the better it is for your body.

By mastering these elements—portion control, meal timing, and label reading—you equip yourself not only to stick to the carb cycling system but also to make choices that enhance your overall health. Eating then becomes an act of nourishment and a pleasure, a balanced dance between fulfilling the body's needs and enjoying the vast array of foods life has to offer. This balance is not just a temporary phase but a sustainable practice, pivotal to maintaining long-term fitness and wellness.

CHAPTER 3: MEAL PLANNING AND PREPARATION

Embarking on a journey of healthy eating with carb cycling is akin to charting a path through a lush, unexplored forest—thrilling yet filled with unknowns. Meal planning and preparation are your compass and map, vital tools to navigate this terrain with confidence. Without them, one might find themselves lost, or worse, reverting to old habits that lead back to square one.

Imagine waking up on a crisp Monday morning with a clear plan—you know exactly what's on today's menu, and the ingredients are ready in your kitchen. This is not a rare, serendipitous occurrence but the result of a well-thought-out strategy laid out in the preceding weekend. Meal planning isn't merely deciding what to eat; it's about creating a flow for your week that aligns with your energy levels, work schedule, and social commitments.

Now, consider the art of meal preparation, which transforms planning on paper into actionable, ready-to-eat meals. It's a Sunday afternoon, and the kitchen buzzes with the sound of chopping vegetables, simmering pots, and perhaps even some upbeat music to make the process enjoyable. This isn't just about cooking—it's a deliberate act of setting yourself up for success. Each container of prepped ingredients is a step closer to your goals. It ensures that when life throws unexpected challenges at you—a last-minute meeting, a child's soccer practice running late—you're armed and ready, with healthy meals that support your carb cycling journey.

Think about how empowering it feels to have control over your dietary intake, to no longer feel at the whim of takeaway menus or office vending machines. With a week's worth of meals planned and prepped, you walk into each day with a sense of preparedness and peace. It's transformative, not just for your body, but for your mind too.

This chapter dives deep into the how and why of effective meal planning and the best practices for meal preparation that even the busiest individual can integrate into their routine. The aim is to equip you with techniques that make your health goals achievable and sustainable, turning what could be a mundane chore into a dynamic part of your wellness journey.

1. CREATING A MEAL PLAN

Creating a meal plan is akin to drafting a personal roadmap for your dietary journey—where each meal aligns not only with your weight loss ambitions but also with the rhythms of your daily life. To embark on this process effectively, start by understanding your body's needs, setting a structure to your meals, and smarter grocery shopping—each a pillar that supports the foundation of your carb cycling success.

Assessing Your Needs

The first step in crafting a meal plan that sticks is a clear evaluation of your personal and health needs. This self-assessment goes beyond knowing your favorite dishes; it involves understanding your body's response to different types of foods, your daily calorie requirements, and how various macronutrients affect your energy and satiety levels.

Recall the days when you felt at your peak, brimming with energy, and identify the meals that helped you there. This reflection guides you to tailor a diet that fits like a glove, ensuring each calorie consumed serves a purpose.

For someone on a carb cycling plan, this assessment takes on multiple dimensions. You'll need to consider the demands of both high-carb and low-carb days. This dual approach ensures your high-carb days fuel intensive physical activities, such as your gym sessions or long runs, while your low-carb days align with lighter, more sedentary periods.

Structuring Your Meals

With a clear understanding of what your body needs, structuring your meals can actually become a creative and enjoyable process. Think of your meal plan as a tapestry, with each thread representing a nutrient tying together to form a vibrant picture of health.

A balanced day on a high-carb day, for example, would paint a picture of hearty whole grains in the morning, a midday splash of legumes or fruits, followed by a dinner rich in fibrous vegetables and a modest serving of protein. On your low-carb days, the palette shifts to proteins and healthy fats, designing meals around lean meats, fish, and generous servings of greens.

However, nutrition should not overshadow enjoyment. The art of carb cycling is crafting meals that are as pleasing to the palate as they are beneficial to the body. Here lies the challenge and the thrill of meal planning. Introduce variety, experiment with herbs and spices, and rotate your protein sources. This not only prevents the dietary monotony that many fear but also ensures a broader intake of nutrients.

Grocery Shopping Tips

Armed with your meal plan, stepping into the supermarket doesn't have to be an overwhelming experience. Efficient and strategic shopping ensures you get everything you need without succumbing to impulse buys that do not serve your goals.

Compile a specific grocery list based on your weekly meal plan: This list becomes your lodestar, guiding you through the aisles and keeping your shopping cart on track. As you jot down your needs, categorize them into produce, proteins, dairy, and so forth. Such organization helps streamline your shopping process, saving you time and preventing the frustration of backtracking for missed items.

Embrace the perimeter: Most grocery stores are designed with fresh foods—produce, dairy, seafood, and meat—lining the walls. Stick to these outer aisles for the bulk of your shopping to naturally avoid the highly processed foods often lurking in the center aisles.

Timing is everything: Schedule your grocery shopping when you're least vulnerable to cravings—generally after meals, when you're satisfied, not when you're starving and everything looks tempting. Moreover, fewer crowds can reduce stress and allow you to focus more on your healthy choices.

Seasonal and local are your friends: Opt for fruits and vegetables that are in season. They're not only fresher and more nutritious but often cheaper too. Plus, supporting local markets ensures a lower carbon footprint, aligning your diet choices with environmental stewardship.

This structured approach to creating a meal plan isn't just about eating right; it's about transforming your relationship with food. It turns meal preparation from a chore into an act of self-care, ensuring each bite not only brings you closer to your weight goals but also builds a foundation for lasting health. As you become more adept at assessing your needs, structuring your meals, and shopping efficiently, you'll find your carb cycling plan doesn't just fit your lifestyle—it enhances it. Each step, from kitchen to table, becomes a testament to living a life brimming with health, vitality, and enjoyment.

2. MEAL PREP STRATEGIES

Once the pathfinding phase of meal planning is complete, the next vital step in our nutritional expedition is meal prep. Consider meal preparation as setting the stage before the main event. Here, our primary goals are efficiency, longevity, and ease, ensuring that healthy eating fits seamlessly into your busy lifestyle. Each strategy—whether it involves batch cooking, proper food storage, or quick prep tips—aims to save you time while maintaining the nutritional integrity of every meal you consume.

Starting with batch cooking, we embrace the philosophy of 'cook once, eat multiple times.' The beauty of this approach lies in its ability to transform a single, dedicated block of cooking time into an array of meals for the days ahead. For instance, roasting a large tray of chicken breasts, cooking a big pot of quinoa, or simmering a batch of your favorite stew does more than just fill your home with enticing aromas—it sets you up for nutritional success. This method not only helps to streamline your week but also opens up more leisure time to spend with family or to unwind.

However, cooking in bulk is only as effective as your ability to store and reheat without losing freshness or flavor. The trick lies in understanding the nuances of food storage. Tupperware and similar food storage containers can be your allies here, but knowing what goes where in the fridge can make a difference. For instance, cooked meats should be stored in the coldest part of the refrigerator to extend their freshness. Grains like rice or quinoa can be kept in airtight containers and used as bases for various dishes throughout the week. By mastering these subtle arts, you ensure that your meals retain their allure, tempting you to stick to your healthy eating plan rather than straying toward less wholesome quick fixes.

Storing cooked meals brings us to another critical aspect of meal prep—reheating. Safe reheating is paramount to maintaining both the nutritional value and safety of food. Each dish has its own ideal method of reheating. For example, steamed vegetables are best reheated over the stove to keep them from turning mushy, while stews and soups can be brought back to life over a gentle heat, which allows flavors to meld even beautifully.

Lastly, not every meal prep session needs to turn into a culinary marathon. Quick and easy strategies can also play a critical role in your diet, especially on unusually hectic days. Have a variety of healthy non-perishables like canned beans, pre-cooked lentils, or instant oats at hand.

These can be lifesavers, providing the backbone for a nutritious meal within minutes. Pair them with fresh produce and some pre-cooked proteins, and you can whip up meals that are not just quick but also well-rounded and satisfying.

Consider smoothie packs, for example—an assortment of frozen fruits, vegetables, protein powder, and perhaps some nuts, all pre-packed into single servings. On a busy morning, all you need to do is blend the contents with a liquid of your choice, and voilà, breakfast is served. Or think about the leftovers strategically. A bit of extra grilled chicken from dinner can become part of a hearty salad for lunch the next day, proving that "quick" can still be nutritious and delicious.

In essence, successful meal prep is less about rigid culinary disciplines and more about smart, sensible cooking practices that align with your lifestyle. By employing these strategies, you convert what might initially appear as a weekly chore into a rhythm that resonates harmoniously with your routine, making healthy dieting a natural part of your daily life.

This intentional approach to meal preparation not only simplifies following the carb cycling plan but also reinforces your commitment to a healthier lifestyle, paving the way for lasting change that extends well beyond mere weight loss. Each step you take in preparing your meals is a step toward a more controlled and conscious way of eating—a true revolution in your kitchen, with effects that ripple through every area of your life.

3. EATING OUT AND SOCIAL SITUATIONS

Navigating the social seas of dining out and attending gatherings while sticking to a carb cycling plan may initially seem like an overbearing challenge. Yet this journey need not be restrictive nor isolating. With the right strategies, you can enjoy the vibrancy of social gatherings or the culinary delights at restaurants without steering off your path towards a healthier lifestyle.

When dining out, the menu, a vast ocean of choices, could either be your ally or adversary. The trick lies in mastering the art of making smart choices. It begins with a pre-visit strategy—most restaurants now offer their menus online. Taking a few moments to review the menu before stepping out helps set your intentions clear and keeps surprises at bay. When selecting dishes, steer towards grilled, baked, steamed, or broiled options—cooking methods that typically imply less oil and unhidden calories compared to their fried or sautéed counterparts. If the menu day is a high-carb day, look for wholesome, fiber-rich carb sources like whole grains; on a low-carb day, focus on proteins and healthy fats. Here's an added tool: don't hesitate to ask for customizations. Most chefs appreciate dietary conscientiousness and can often swap out certain ingredients for a plate that better suits your dietary plan.

Beyond the personal plate decisions, consider the setting. A table away from the kitchen might minimize spontaneous decisions spurred by the sights and smells of tantalizing dishes.

Another effective tactic is to be the first to order, setting a healthy tone that might subtly influence your dining companions. This proactivity ensures you dictate your meal course, not the ambiance or the preferences of others.

Turning to social gatherings, these events can often seem like a notorious pitfall—a buffet of temptations. Whether it's a family barbecue or a friend's birthday, the best approach is a blend of preparedness and flexibility. If possible, contribute a dish to share. This not only guarantees that there will be at least one healthy item available, but it also introduces others to your lifestyle, creating an opportunity for support and understanding. When faced with an array of unknown dishes, fill your plate with vegetables and proteins first—this both adheres to carb cycling principles and reduces room for more indulgent choices.

Moreover, focus on the social aspect, not just the eating. Engaging in conversation or participating in activities can divert attention from purely food-focused interactions. If you opt for a drink, choices like a glass of dry wine or a light beer are preferable, considering moderation.

For those who travel, whether for work or leisure, staying true to a meal plan could seem daunting. Yet, travel-friendly food options are more accessible today than ever before. Convenience can align with compliance if planned right. Packing non-perishable snacks like nuts, seeds, protein bars (low in sugar), or even canned fish can act as quick fixes when healthy options are scarce. When selecting accommodations, consider places with a kitchenette or at least a refrigerator, giving you the flexibility to store some basic groceries or meal prep items. Many local supermarkets offer pre-cut fresh vegetables, rotisserie chickens, and wholesome salad options, which can be conveniently assembled into meals.

Moreover, leveraging technology can ease your culinary ventures in unfamiliar territories. Apps dedicated to restaurant reviews and healthy food recommendations can be invaluable in locating dining spots that align with your dietary preferences.

By embracing these strategies, eating out, attending social events, or traveling doesn't have to be a deviation from your carb cycling journey—you can control your diet without social sacrifice, harnessing the joy and connectivity these experiences bring. This adaptability not only makes your diet approach sustainable over the long term but also integrates health into every dimension of your life, making every meal an extension of your commitment to wellness, whether at home or on the go.

CHAPTER 4: OVERCOMING CHALLENGES

Embarking on a journey toward better health and weight loss is akin to setting sail on vast, uncharted waters. It brings excitement and hope, but unavoidable storms and challenges also appear on the horizon. In the realm of carb cycling and transformative diets, these challenges manifest as cravings, motivational dips, and frustrating plateaus. Addressing these issues is not just a part of the journey; it's essential for reaching the destination.

As we delve into the complexities of navigating dietary and emotional challenges, it's important to recognize that each struggle is a stepping stone towards greater self-awareness and control. Think of managing cravings not just as resisting temptations, but as an opportunity to understand deeper emotional and physical signals. When cravings hit, they often carry hidden messages about our needs for comfort, stress relief, or even entertainment—decoding these messages can turn mindless eating into mindful understanding.

Staying motivated can feel particularly tough on days when the scale doesn't budge or when life's demands pull us in multiple directions. Here, the key is to anchor your daily actions to deeper values and long-term visions. Why does this journey matter to you? What will you gain by staying on this path? These are questions worth revisiting regularly. Each small step, each healthy meal, and each resisted urge is a triumph that cumulatively leads to significant changes.

Encountering a plateau can be disheartening—seeing little or no results despite your best efforts. However, this stage is an almost inevitable phase of any weight loss journey and an indicator to reassess and recalibrate. It is not the body's stubborn refusal to change but a sign that it's time for new strategies in diet or exercise routines.

Navigating through these challenges requires a blend of science-backed strategies and personal introspection, transforming potential setbacks into opportunities for growth and learning. Remember, the journey through carb cycling is as much about building resilience and learning about your body as it is about losing weight. Each challenge overcome doesn't just bring you closer to your goal weight but also to becoming a more empowered and self-aware individual.

1. MANAGING CRAVINGS AND EMOTIONAL EATING

In our daily lives, emotional eating and cravings often appear as saboteurs on our journey to health and weight loss. They sneak up on us during moments of vulnerability, offering comfort in the form of food when what we really need might be a listening ear or a restful pause. Understanding and managing these impulses are crucial because they not only interfere with our dietary plans but also affect our emotional well-being.

Identifying Triggers

The first step towards mastering cravings and emotional eating is to recognize the triggers. Triggers are like silent alarms that go off in response to different situations or emotions. For many, stress is a significant trigger.

It could be the stress from a looming deadline at work or an ongoing conflict in a personal relationship. Others might find boredom or feelings of loneliness as the catalysts for heading towards the pantry.

Start by keeping a 'trigger journal.' Every time you find yourself craving a snack outside your meal plan or indulging more than usual, jot down what was happening or how you were feeling at that moment. Over time, patterns will emerge, and you will be able to identify which situations or emotions prompt you to turn to food. This awareness is a powerful tool; it gives you the chance to handle the trigger before it leads to a craving.

Strategies to Combat Cravings

Once you know your triggers, you can develop strategies to combat cravings. If stress is a trigger, find stress-reduction techniques that work for you, such as meditation, yoga, or simply taking a brisk walk to clear your mind. If boredom makes you eat, try to engage in activities that keep you mentally stimulated.

Prepare for inevitable cravings by creating a 'cravings emergency kit.' Fill it with healthier alternatives that satisfy the urge without derailing your diet. For instance, if you crave sweets, a piece of dark chocolate or a fruit might suffice. The key is portion control and choosing an alternative that aligns with your carb cycling plan.

Another effective strategy is the 15-minute rule. When a craving hits, promise yourself to wait 15 minutes before giving in. During that time, engage in a distraction like reading a book or calling a friend. Often, the craving will pass, and you will have successfully avoided an unnecessary indulgence.

Mindful Eating Techniques

Mindful eating is about creating a deep connection with your food by engaging all the senses, understanding the source of your cravings, and learning to distinguish between true hunger and emotional hunger. This practice not only helps in managing weight but also enhances the enjoyment of your meals.

Start by eating slowly and without distractions. Avoid eating while watching TV or scrolling through your smartphone. Instead, focus on the texture, smell, and flavor of your food. This helps in recognizing when you're full, reducing the likelihood of overeating.

Question your hunger. Before you reach for a snack, ask yourself if you are really hungry or just responding to an emotion or situation. Imagine eating something healthy like an apple or a vegetable; if that doesn't seem appealing, you're likely not genuinely hungry.

Engage in regular check-ins with yourself. How do you feel about your food choices? Are you eating out of hunger or habit? These questions can help foster a healthier eating attitude and prevent automatic responses to eat under stress or other emotional states.

Through the identification of triggers, strategic combat against cravings, and the adoption of mindful eating practices, you can overtake emotional eating and transform your relationship with food. It isn't about denying yourself pleasure; it's about finding a balance that satisfies both your body and soul, which is essential for lasting success in any health and weight management journey. By addressing these aspects, you are not just dieting—you are revising your lifestyle for long-term wellness and joy in nourishment.

2. STAYING MOTIVATED

Embarking on a weight loss journey with carb cycling is akin to running a marathon. It requires persistence, patience, and plenty of motivation to keep going even when the finish line seems distant. Staying motivated can be challenging, especially during periods when progress slows down or life gets overwhelmingly busy. However, keeping that spark of motivation alive is crucial for long-term success and transformation.

Setting Short-Term Milestones

One of the most effective ways to maintain motivation is by setting short-term milestones. These are like mini-goals that are easier to achieve and keep you focused on the progress you're making. Instead of setting one large goal, break it down into smaller, manageable parts. For instance, instead of focusing solely on losing 30 pounds, set a milestone to lose the first five pounds. Then set another for increasing your vegetable intake each day, or reducing processed food gradually.

These short-term goals should be specific, measurable, achievable, relevant, and time-bound (SMART). An example might be, "In the next two weeks, I will replace dessert with a healthy alternative at least five days a week." This kind of goal isn't just about reducing calorie intake; it's about creating a sustainable healthy habit, which is far more beneficial in the long run.

Celebrating Small Wins

Every milestone achieved is a win and should be celebrated. Celebrating is an essential part of the motivation cycle because it reinforces the positive behavior that led to the success. However, the key is to celebrate in a way that doesn't undermine your progress. For instance, rewarding yourself for losing the first five pounds with a big slice of cake might be counterproductive. Instead, consider rewards that align with your new lifestyle, such as buying a new workout outfit or treating yourself to a professional massage.

Celebrations do not always have to involve spending money. They can be as simple as taking a day off for yourself to relax and enjoy your favorite activities without feeling rushed. The point is to acknowledge your hard work and allow yourself to enjoy the fruits of your labor in a way that supports your continued success.

Building a Support System

Weight loss and lifestyle changes can be lonely journeys if you're walking them alone. Hence, it's crucial to build a support system. This could mean different things for different people.

For some, it may be family members who cheer you on, while for others, it might be friends or colleagues who are also on their own health journeys.

Joining a community, whether online or in-person, that focuses on healthy living can provide emotional support, motivation, and accountability. For example, participating in a local walking group or joining a carb cycling forum online can connect you with individuals facing similar challenges. Such interactions can provide new insights, celebrate successes, and share strategies for overcoming obstacles.

Furthermore, consider finding a buddy or a mentor who has been through a similar journey. They can provide valuable guidance, tips, and a much-needed empathetic ear. Just be sure that this network is encouraging and aligned with the healthy habits you are trying to cultivate.

In such supportive settings, it's also valuable to reciprocate; being someone else's cheerleader can reinforce your own commitment. It's a circle of motivation that keeps all members moving forward. Also, verbalizing your goals to your support group can increase your accountability drastically, making you more likely to stick with your plans.

By setting short-term milestones, celebrating small wins appropriately, and building a strong support system, staying motivated on a carb cycling plan becomes more manageable and even enjoyable. These strategies aren't just about keeping you on track; they're about transforming the journey itself into a rewarding and enriching experience. After all, the ultimate goal is not just to lose weight but to live a healthier, more vibrant life.

3. DEALING WITH PLATEAUS

Hitting a weight loss plateau can be one of the most frustrating parts of anyone's health journey. You're following your carb cycling plan, you're exercising, and initially, you saw great results. But suddenly, progress stalls; the scales won't budge, and it feels like your efforts are getting you nowhere. This is what we call a plateau, and it's a natural part of the weight loss process. Understanding this, adjusting your approach, and maintaining patience and persistence are key to overcoming it.

Understanding Plateaus

A weight loss plateau occurs when your body adapts to the changes you've made. Initially, especially if you had a significant amount of weight to lose, changes in diet and exercise have a large impact. Your body was not used to these actions, so it responded quickly. However, as you lose weight, your body requires fewer calories to function than it did at a higher weight. That, combined with the possibility that your metabolism might slow down as part of this adjustment, leads to a plateau.

Recognizing a plateau's inevitability is crucial. It is not a sign of failure or a reason to give up. Rather, it's a biological signal from your body, indicating that it's time to mix things up and push through to the next phase of your weight loss journey.

Adjusting Your Carb Cycling Plan

When you hit a plateau, the first action is to reassess and tweak your carb cycling plan. Perhaps your body has gotten too accustomed to the pattern of high and low-carb days. It might be time to alter these patterns. For instance, if you were doing three high-carb days followed by one low-carb day, you might switch to a 2:2 ratio to shock your body into response. Additionally, assess your caloric intake and expenditure. Even subtle changes in food intake or activity levels can restart weight loss.

Another factor might be the types of carbohydrates you're consuming. Quality is as important as quantity. Focus on high-fiber, nutrient-dense carbs like whole grains, vegetables, and fruits and avoid simple sugars and refined carbs. Sometimes, making these small shifts can lead your body out of a plateau.

Staying Patient and Persistent

Patience and persistence are your best allies in battling a plateau. Weight loss is not a linear process; there will be ups and downs, and how you handle these can determine your success. Keep a detailed food and exercise diary to monitor exactly what you're eating and how much you're moving. This documentation can help you and possibly a nutrition professional figure out what changes will help you start losing weight again.

It's also essential to focus on other indicators of health improvement. Maybe the scales haven't moved, but do your clothes fit better? Do you have more energy? Are you sleeping better? Improvements in these areas also signify the continuing success of your health journey.

Remember that weight loss plateaus are temporary. With the right adjustments to your carb cycling plan and a commitment to stay the course, you will be able to continue toward your health and fitness goals. The key is not to get discouraged. Instead, use the plateau as a learning experience about your body and its needs. Adjustments can bring about a greater understanding of nutrition, metabolism, and physical health, contributing to more informed decisions as you move forward.

Navigating through a plateau is more than just an exercise in weight loss—it's a journey in perseverance and learning to commit to your health, irrespective of the challenges. By staying patient, persistent, and proactive in adjusting your strategies, you equip yourself with the tools to not just overcome this plateau but any future challenges as well.

CHAPTER 5: ENHANCING YOUR RESULTS

As you journey through the transformative world of carb cycling, you may reach a point where the thrill of initial weight loss starts to plateau and the novelty of meal planning becomes a regular part of your routine. This is a pivotal moment in your journey, not just to celebrate how far you've come, but also to enhance the results you've worked so hard to achieve. Chapter 5 is dedicated to just that—taking your accomplishments and amplifying them for sustained success.

Imagine carb cycling as a finely tuned orchestra. Initially, each section learns to play its parts, coming together in harmony to perform the symphony of weight loss and improved fitness. But as any musician would tell you, the magic lies not just in playing the notes right but in playing them with passion and precision, continually improving with each performance. Similarly, enhancing your carb cycling results isn't about reinventing your diet but refining and adapting it to keep the music playing sweetly in your life.

Incorporating exercise tailored to your carb intake days transforms your body into a more efficient machine, turning nutrients into energy with the precision of a skilled conductor. Monitoring your progress and making necessary adjustments keeps you attuned to your body's needs, much like a musician tuning their instrument. And perhaps most importantly, preparing for long-term success ensures that this lifestyle change is sustainable, allowing you to dance to the rhythm of good health indefinitely.

As you delve into this chapter, you'll find strategies not merely for maintaining the momentum but for propelling yourself forward. This isn't just about pushing harder; it's about pushing smarter, using the insights gained from your experiences to optimize your approach. Whether it's refining your meal plans, tweaking your workouts, or adjusting your goals, the focus is on fine-tuning the elements that will keep you moving towards a healthier version of yourself. Here, we holistically enhance the melody of your wellness journey, ensuring each note resonates with vitality and vigor.

1. INCORPORATING EXERCISE

Exercise and carb cycling fit together like a lock and key, each enhancing the efficiency of the other. When you incorporate exercise into your carb cycling routine, you're not just burning calories; you're strategically boosting your metabolism and enhancing your body's ability to utilize carbohydrates and fats more effectively. Here, let's explore not only which types of workouts will complement your carb cycling days best but also how you can smartly schedule these activities and understand the pivotal role of rest and recovery.

Firstly, understanding which workouts to pair with your high-carb and low-carb days can make a substantial difference in your results. On high-carb days, your body has a surplus of readily available energy. These are the days to engage in high-intensity workouts such as weight training, sprinting, or high-intensity interval training (HIIT). These types of exercises require quick, explosive bursts of energy, which will utilize the carbohydrates you're consuming. Moreover, strength training significantly contributes to muscle gain, which not only shapes your body but also increases your resting metabolic rate, meaning you'll burn more calories even while at rest.

Conversely, your low-carb days should focus on activities that primarily use fat as an energy source. This is the perfect time for steady-state cardio exercises like jogging, swimming, or cycling. These activities don't demand as much quick energy but require endurance, making them ideal when your intake of carbs is lower. The bonus here is that these types of exercises can also help in reducing stress, improving your overall cardiovascular health, and enhancing mood stabilization — much needed when dietary carbohydrates are limited.

Now, while knowing what workouts to do on specific days is key, equally important is how you schedule these workouts. Your exercise routine should ideally work in harmony with your carb cycling plan. For instance, plan your high-intensity, strength-training sessions on those days when your carb intake is at its peak. This synchronization maximizes glycogen availability, thereby enhancing your performance and recovery. On the days scheduled for low-carb intake, align with lower-intensity, fat-oxidizing cardio workouts. This not only helps in managing energy levels more effectively but also supports fat loss.

Creating a balanced workout schedule involves considering not just the type of exercise but the timing. If you're an early riser, capitalizing on the natural energy boost in the morning could make your high-intensity workouts more effective. Exercising in the morning on a high-carb day could also enhance glucose metabolism throughout the day. On low-carb days, consider scheduling exercises in the later part of the day when your body has adjusted to lower carb levels, ensuring you still can maintain performance without feeling depleted.

Furthermore, the importance of rest and recovery days cannot be overstated. They are just as crucial as your workout days. Recovery is when your muscles repair, grow, and strengthen. Over-exercising without sufficient recovery can lead to fatigue, injuries, and even hinder your progress. On your rest days, it isn't about doing nothing; it's about letting your body recover while doing lighter activities like stretching, yoga, or a leisurely walk. These activities enhance blood flow, which helps in reducing muscle soreness and speeds up the recovery process.

Additionally, align your recovery days with your low-carb intake days. This approach can enhance your body's fat-burning ability while replenishing and repairing muscle tissues. Remember, rest days are integral in ensuring the longevity of your fitness journey. They help maintain a balanced and realistic approach to exercise, which aligns perfectly with the sustainable ethos of carb cycling.

In conclusion, weaving exercise into your carb cycling strategy isn't just about randomly picking workouts and squeezing them into your week. It's about thoughtful alignment of your body's nutritional needs with physical activities that will optimize and enhance your metabolic responses. By planning your exercises around your carb intake, attuning to your body's cues, and ensuring adequate recovery, you pave the way not just for effective weight loss, but for a holistic, energized, and sustainable fitness journey. This blend of smart eating and exercising leads to not just looking good, but feeling phenomenal. And isn't that the ultimate goal of any health transformation journey?

2. MONITORING AND ADJUSTING

Embarking on a journey of transformation is commendable, but the true magic lies in your ability to adapt and fine-tune your strategies based on real-world results. The cycle of monitoring and adjusting your diet and exercise routine is fundamental to this journey. This not only helps you stay on track but also empowers you to make informed decisions that propel you towards your health and fitness goals more effectively.

Let's delve into the practice of keeping a food and exercise journal, a potent tool that might initially seem cumbersome but proves to be invaluable. Documenting your daily intake of food and noting down details about your exercise regime provides you with a clear overview of your habits — both good and bad. This practice allows you to reflect on what you're actually consuming versus what you think you're consuming and also to track the consistency and intensity of your workouts.

Moreover, a journal acts as a mirror, reflecting your patterns that typically go unnoticed. For instance, you might discover through consistent logging that your energy levels dip after consuming certain foods, or that you tend to skip your workout routines on days when your carb intake is at its lowest. Recognizing such patterns is crucial for making effective adjustments. It's about becoming a detective in your own life, uncovering clues that lead to a better understanding of your body's responses.

Now, let's talk about analyzing your results from the journal. This isn't about skimming through the pages for general insights but involves a deeper analysis to gather actionable data. Each week, take some time to review your entries for insights on what's propelling you towards your goals and what's holding you back. It might be helpful to note trends such as weight fluctuations, energy levels, mood changes, and other health markers like sleep quality and digestion. Connecting these dots can often highlight the subtle impacts of dietary choices and exercise habits.

Analyzing such data enables you to understand the effectiveness of your current carb cycling plan and workout regimen. Perhaps your journal indicates that your low-carb days are too intense and coincide with high-stress periods, suggesting a need for realignment. Or maybe during high-carb days, you're not exercising enough to justify the increased calorie intake. These are the types of insights that can drive substantial improvements in your diet and exercise protocols.

Once you have gathered and analyzed your data, the next step is to make the necessary adjustments. This should be approached with a mindset of experimentation. Small, incremental changes allow you to test different strategies and see how they impact your results. For example, if you find you're often fatigued, you might adjust your carb cycling to include a moderate increase in carbs on specific days to see if it boosts your energy levels. Similarly, if weight loss plateaus, introducing an additional day of high-intensity training might reignite your metabolic rate.

Adjustments should also reflect improvements in your physical fitness and dietary responses over time. As your body adapts and your fitness levels increase, your needs will change. This might mean recalibrating your macronutrient ratios or introducing more complex exercises to continue challenging your body. Keep in mind, the goal of these adjustments is not to overhaul your entire plan but to refine it so it continues to align with your evolving objectives.

Lastly, remember that monitoring and adjusting is an ongoing process. You're not setting a new plan in stone but iterating on your lifestyle habits. Periodical revisitation of your journal and analysis will be essential as you progress. Consider setting monthly check-ins with yourself to review your journal, assess your satisfaction with your progress, and make necessary adjustments. It's similar to a business reviewing its quarterly results; the aim is to see what's working, what isn't, and how the strategy can be adapted for better results in the next period.

By making the monitoring and adjustment process a regular part of your health routine, you turn passive experiences into active experiments where learning and growth lead to continued success. This methodical approach ensures that your journey in carb cycling and exercise will be dynamic and responsive, adapting to meet your body's needs and your personal goals. In this way, you're not only pursuing better health, you're mastering it.

3. LONG-TERM SUCCESS

Navigating the path to weight loss and improved fitness is akin to climbing a mountain. Reaching the summit is exhilarating—symbolizing the achievement of your goals—but the journey doesn't end there. The descent, or the maintenance phase, requires as much strategy and care as the ascent. This final phase of your carb cycling adventure is about transitioning into long-term maintenance, establishing sustainable habits, and preventing weight regain.

The transition from 'active weight loss' to 'maintenance' in your diet is a critical shift that affects not only how you eat but how you perceive your lifestyle changes. It's the moment when dieting stops being about losing weight and starts focusing on sustaining the healthy body and habits you've developed. To make this transition effectively, start by gradually increasing your carb intake, raising it to a level that maintains your weight rather than reduces it. It's about finding that new equilibrium where your calorie intake matches your output without leading to weight gain.

Part of this balancing act involves listening to your body's signals—a skill that you've honed meticulously by this point in your journey. You might notice, for instance, that certain carb levels make you feel more energized, while others may cause sluggishness or discomfort. Use these cues to adjust your intake so that you're nourished and satiated, without overtipping the scales.

As you stabilize your carb intake, also begin to shift your goal-setting focus. While initial targets were likely centered around weight loss metrics, maintenance goals should prioritize strength, flexibility, cardiovascular health, and emotional well-being. This might mean setting objectives like improving your time on a 5k run, mastering a new yoga pose, or meditating daily. Goals in the maintenance phase should be about enhancing your life quality and celebrating what your body can do.

Now, cultivating sustainable habits is key to ensuring that your maintenance phase doesn't revert into old patterns. Sustainability is not just about adhering to specific dietary rules. It's about creating an environment where these rules are easy, satisfying, and beneficial to follow. For instance, continuation in meal planning and prep that you've learned should not stop once the weight loss phase is over.

They should evolve into more flexible practices that still maintain a structure but allow for greater variability and spontaneity—this could mean planning meals around seasonal produce or trying new cuisines to keep your diet exciting and culturally enriching.

Physical activity should also remain a cornerstone of your daily routine. Now is the time to explore new sports or activities that might have seemed daunting before. Joining a local hiking group, taking up dance classes, or even engaging in more community-oriented activities like volunteer gardening can keep physical activity enjoyable and integrated into your social life.

Furthermore, community engagement and social support networks are invaluable. Continuing to share your journey, challenges, and successes with supportive peers or groups can provide motivation and accountability. Whether it's through online communities, local fitness groups, or simply a group of friends, maintaining social ties within a supportive environment can greatly enhance your long-term adherence to your healthy lifestyle.

Lastly, an important aspect of long-term success is vigilance against weight regain. This doesn't mean obsessively monitoring the scale but being aware of how fluctuations in your body's weight and composition can signal the need for slight adjustments in diet or activity. Regular, non-obsessive monitoring—a quick check every week or bi-weekly—can help you catch and address minor gains before they become larger issues.

Also, understand that life will throw challenges at you—stressful periods at work, family responsibilities, holidays, and so on. Each of these can potentially disrupt your routine. Prepare strategies in advance for these times. This may include having a set of baseline minimum workouts for particularly busy weeks or a list of healthy stress-reduction techniques like deep-breathing exercises or quick meditations.

In essence, the maintenance phase is about integrating the principles of carb cycling and healthy living into a flexible, enjoyable, and sustainable lifestyle. It's not about clinging tightly to the rules but about adapting them to enhance your life's quality, ensuring that this journey leaves a lasting impact on your overall wellness. Remember, the true success of your transformation lies not just in the pounds you've lost but in the habits you've gained and the assurance that you can maintain this healthier, happier version of yourself.

CHAPTER 6: THE ULTIMATE 3 MEAL PLANS METHOD

Welcome to a transformative journey with "The Ultimate 3 Meal Plans Method." If you've ever felt lost in the myriad of nutrition advice and diet plans, this chapter is about to simplify your path to effective weight loss. This method isn't just about shedding pounds; it's about crafting a relationship with food that feels as natural and sustaining as breathing.

Imagine starting your mornings knowing exactly what's on your plate - each meal tailored not just to fuel your body, but to coax it gently towards fat loss, increased energy, and greater overall health. The beauty of the 3 Meal Plans Method lies in its structure and adaptability to your life's pace. Whether you're a busy parent juggling schedules or a professional trying to balance work and wellness, this approach bends to fit your day, not the other way around.

Through the next pages, we will dive into a three-phase meal planning system that gradually adjusts carbs, rather than eliminating them abruptly. This is where the art of carb cycling truly comes to play—high-carb days to boost your metabolism and support intense workouts, low-carb days to promote fat burning, and medium-carb days to maintain and balance. Think of it as tuning a musical instrument; each adjustment brings you closer to the sweet spot of harmony.

Let's take the guesswork out of meal planning. Each meal plan spans two weeks, giving your body the necessary time to adapt, respond, and thrive. You will be guided through each step, with detailed daily meal breakdowns that don't just satisfy your taste buds but also advance you towards your goals. And it's not just about the lists of foods; it's about understanding why these choices propel you forward in your fitness journey.

As we explore these meal plans, remember, this is more than a diet. It's a stepping stone toward a sustainable lifestyle. A lifestyle where you don't just live, but flourish.

1. INTRODUCTION TO THE 3 MEAL PLANS

Embarking on a carb cycling journey can sometimes feel like setting sail on open waters — the promise of discovery is thrilling, but the vastness can be overwhelming. My breakthrough is to demystify this process through the "3 Meal Plans Method," an approach designed to introduce a gradual reduction in carbohydrates, gradually steering you toward a healthier, leaner life without the shock and rebound associated with extreme dietary changes.

The Concept of Gradual Carb Reduction

The central thesis of this method is straightforward: rather than drastically cutting carbohydrates from your diet, we reduce them gradually. Think of your typical diet as a staircase. On a standard diet, you might be a few steps higher in carbohydrate intake. Each phase of this method acts as a step down, easing your body into a new metabolic state. This gradual descent helps manage insulin levels and maintains metabolic balance, ensuring your body can efficiently switch from using carbs to fats as its primary fuel source.

This gradual reduction helps curb the common pitfalls of traditional diets, such as intense hunger and the inevitable carb cravings that sabotage long-term compliance and success. It gives your body the time to adapt to each new level of carbohydrate intake, which can significantly enhance your metabolic flexibility — your body's ability to switch between burning carbs and fats efficiently. This approach not only makes the dietary transition smoother but also minimizes the stress and shock to your system, paving the way for sustainable weight loss and health benefits.

Benefits of the 3 Meal Plan Method

Delving into the benefits, the 3 Meal Plan Method extends beyond simple weight loss. The strategic variation in carbohydrate intake across different days maximizes fat burning while maintaining high energy levels — a rarity in low-carb diet plans where sluggishness and fatigue can often take hold.

1. **Sustained Energy Levels:** By cycling your carbohydrate intake, you ensure that your body receives enough fuel on high-carb days to perform energetically in workouts and daily activities, while low-carb days heighten your body's ability to tap into fat stores for energy.

2. **Enhanced Metabolic Health:** Gradual carb reduction can enhance insulin sensitivity, a pinnacle of metabolic health. This sensitivity facilitates better blood sugar management, which is crucial for reducing the risk of diabetes and other metabolic syndromes.

3. **Flexible Dietary Structure:** The structure of the meal plans welcomes spontaneity. Life is unpredictable, and this system is designed to adapt to late-night work schedules, unexpected family dinners, and last-minute changes that would throw a rigid diet off balance.

4. **Psychological Ease:** Less abrupt change means less mental and emotional resistance. The psychological aspect of eating - your connection and attitude towards food - plays an enormous role in the success of any diet. Gradual change fosters a more positive and sustainable relationship with food.

5. **Customizable and Family-Friendly:** These meal plans are tailored to suit not just the lone individual but families as well. Recipes and meal ideas can often be adjusted for portion sizes, making it an inclusive approach for household meal planning.

How to Use the Meal Plans

Using the meal plans involves more than following recipes; it's about understanding your body's responses to different types of foods and learning to adjust portions and ingredients to better meet your dietary needs. Each two-week meal plan serves as a guide and template, not a strict rule book.

- **Start with Assessment:** Before you dive into the first meal plan, take a week to assess your current eating habits. Note things like your energy levels, typical intake of carbs, and how you feel physically and emotionally throughout the day.

- **Phase Introduction:** Each phase should be entered gently. Begin by integrating the suggested meals slowly, replacing your usual meals one at a time. This might seem like a slow start, but it builds a solid foundation for the changes to come.

- **Tailor Your Portions:** Depending on your daily calorie needs — which vary based on sex, age, activity level, and personal goals — you may need to adjust the portion sizes. The plans offer flexibility to scale recipes up for a family setting or down for fewer people.

- **Check-In Regularly:** At the end of each two-week period, evaluate what's working and what's not. Are you often hungry? Do you feel more energized? Use this feedback to tweak the upcoming meal plans to better suit your needs.

- **Be Mindful of Changes:** As you progress through each phase, take note of both the physical and psychological changes. Are certain days harder than others? Are there meals that you look forward to? Insights like these can help adapt the meal plans to be more enjoyable and effective.

By the end of the six weeks, you will not only have navigated through three different carb intake levels but also learned how to adapt a meal plan to your changing lifestyle and needs. You'll be equipped not just with recipes, but with the understanding of how to modify them to continue sustaining your progress independently, turning carb cycling into a sustainable lifestyle rather than a finite diet.

This method isn't just about what you eat; it's about transforming your relationship with food to one where you are in control, leading to a healthier, happier you.

2. MEAL PLAN 1: WEEKS 1-2

Welcome to the initial phase of your carb cycling journey! The first two weeks are pivotal, setting the tone for your adventure into mindful, strategic eating. Here in Meal Plan 1, you'll gently start transitioning from your usual carbohydrate intake to slightly lower levels, without overwhelming your system or sacrificing satisfaction at the dining table. Let's break down this introductory phase to make every meal an easy step toward your weight loss goals.

DAY	BREAKFAST	LUNCH	SNACK	DINNER
1	Classic Vanilla Oatmeal with Fresh Berries	Tropical Quinoa and Black Bean Salad	Berry Almond Smoothie Bowl	Mediterranean Whole Wheat Pasta Primavera
2	Banana and Almond Butter Smoothie	Chicken Shawarma Brown Rice Bowl (reduce rice portion)	Greek Yogurt with Nuts and Seeds	Herb-Crusted Chicken Breast with Steamed Vegetables
3	Spirited Raspberry Chia Oatmeal	Turkey and Quinoa Stuffed Peppers	Fig and Pistachio Greek Yogurt Parfait	Baked Cod with Roasted Vegetables
4	Golden Turmeric Oatmeal	Mediterranean Quinoa and Black Bean Salad	Nutty Banana Blender Pancakes	Lemon Garlic Shrimp and Whole Wheat Pasta Primavera
5	Spicy Banana Almond Shake	Grilled Veggie and Hummus Wrap (reduce wrap portion)	Mixed Nuts and Seeds	Cauliflower Rice with Shrimp
6	Matcha Berry Parfait with Greek Yogurt	Southwest Turkey and Quinoa Stuffed Peppers	Blueberry Buckwheat Pancakes	Spaghetti Squash with Marinara and Meatballs
7	Berry Almond Overnight Oats	Spirited Raspberry Chia Oatmeal	Tropical Mango-Papaya Smoothie Bowl	Thai Basil Chicken and Brown Rice Stir-Fry
8	Vanilla Chai Greek Yogurt Parfaits	Mediterranean Grilled Veggie and Hummus Wrap (reduce wrap portion)	Veggie Sticks with Hummus	Beef and Broccoli Stir-Fry
9	Nutty Banana Blender Pancakes	Chicken and Pearl Barley Soup with Root Vegetables	Fig and Pistachio Greek Yogurt Parfait	Turkey Chili
10	Spirited Raspberry Chia Oatmeal	Salmon Quinoa Pilaf with Asparagus	Tropical Quinoa and Black Bean Salad	Whole Wheat Pasta Primavera with Grilled Vegetables
11	Spicy Banana Almond Shake	Chicken Shawarma Brown Rice Bowl (reduce rice portion)	Greek Yogurt and Berry Cups	Cauliflower Rice with Shrimp
12	Banana and Almond Butter Smoothie	Chicken and Barley Soup with Mushrooms	Mediterranean Quinoa and Black Bean Salad	Baked Cod with Roasted Vegetables
13	Berry Almond Overnight Oats	Spring Vegetable Whole Wheat Pasta Primavera	Tropical Mango-Papaya Smoothie Bowl	Lemon Garlic Shrimp and Whole Wheat Pasta Primavera

14	Vanilla Chai Greek Yogurt Parfaits	Zucchini Noodles with Pesto and Chicken	Mixed Nuts and Seeds	Herb-Crusted Chicken Breast with Steamed Vegetables

Tips for Success

1. **Prep in Advance:** Spend a little time on Sunday prepping parts of meals for the week. Chop vegetables, cook grains like quinoa or brown rice in bulk, and portion out snack foods like almonds and cheese. This makes putting meals together much faster and easier during the busy week.
2. **Stay Hydrated:** Sometimes, thirst is mistaken for hunger. Make sure you're drinking plenty of water throughout the day, which can help with digestion and overall energy levels.
3. **Listen to Your Body:** As you adjust your carb intake, be mindful of how you feel. If a meal leaves you feeling sluggish or still hungry, consider adjusting portions or ingredients in future meals. Tailoring the diet to your personal needs is crucial for long-term success.
4. **Stay Flexible:** Don't be too hard on yourself if a meal or a day doesn't go exactly as planned. This journey is about overall trends, not perfection. If you indulge a bit more at a certain meal, balance it out with lighter options later on.
5. **Involve Your Household:** If you're preparing meals for more than just yourself, involve your family or roommates in the meal planning and preparation. Meals that appeal to the whole household are more likely to become a part of your regular routine, making it easier to stick to your new eating plan.
6. **Keep a Journal:** Tracking what you eat, how you feel, and your physical activity can be extremely insightful as you move through the phases of carb cycling. Use this journal as a tool to connect the dots between your diet, your energy levels, and your mood.

Meal Plan 1 is designed to gently acclimatize you to a new way of thinking about carbs and their place in a balanced diet. As you move through these first two weeks, keep an open mind, and remember that each meal is a building block towards a more energized, streamlined, and healthier you. Enjoy the journey to discovering how simple tweaks to your eating habits can make a profound difference in how you feel and look.

3. MEAL PLAN 2: WEEKS 3-4

As you transition into Weeks 3-4 of your carb cycling journey with Meal Plan 2, you'll notice the structure of your meals shift slightly as we continue the gradual reduction of carbohydrates. This phase is designed to deepen the work started in the first two weeks, enhancing fat metabolism while maintaining muscle mass and fullness throughout the day.

DAY	BREAKFAST	LUNCH	SNACK	DINNER
1	Tropical Yogurt Delight	Turkey and Quinoa Stuffed Peppers with Sundried Tomatoes and Goat Cheese	Spiced Orange Oatmeal Cookies	Herbed Baked Salmon with Citrus Quinoa
2	Savory Avocado Toast with Poached Egg and Arugula	Spicy Thai Peanut Veggie Wrap (reduce wrap portion)	Avocado Lime Hummus with Herbed Veggie Sticks	Colorful Veggie Stir-Fry with Tofu and Cashews
3	Pistachio and Matcha Greek Yogurt Delight	Quinoa-Stuffed Baked Salmon	Berry Nut Yogurt Fiesta	Spaghetti Squash with Marinara and Turkey Meatballs

4	Caprese Avocado Toast with Soft Boiled Egg	Turkey and Quinoa Stuffed Peppers with Feta and Spinach	Tropical Twist Oatmeal Cookies	Baked Cod with Roasted Rainbow Carrots and Parsnips
5	Egg-ocado Toast with Cherry Tomatoes and Feta	California Avocado and Sprouts Wrap (reduce wrap portion)	Spicy Tamari Trail Mix	Braised Spaghetti Squash with Chermoula and Crumbled Feta
6	Savory Spinach and Feta Whole Grain Pancakes	Sweet Potato and Kale Stir-Fry	Berry Lavender Greek Yogurt Cups	Turkey and Veggie Chili
7	Pomegranate and Walnut Parfait with Greek Yogurt	Mediterranean Veggie and Chickpea Sauté	Classic Chewy Oatmeal Raisin Cookies	Miso Glazed Spaghetti Squash with Sesame Seeds
8	Savory Avocado Toast with Poached Egg and Arugula	Sun-Dried Tomato and Almond Pesto Zucchini Noodles	Avocado Lime Hummus with Herbed Veggie Sticks	Spicy Shrimp Over Lime Infused Cauliflower Rice
9	Pistachio and Matcha Greek Yogurt Delight	Turkey and Quinoa Stuffed Peppers with Feta and Spinach	Spicy Tamari Trail Mix	Classic Turkey Chili
10	Pomegranate and Walnut Parfait with Greek Yogurt	Mediterranean Veggie and Chickpea Sauté	Tropical Twist Oatmeal Cookies	Herbed Baked Salmon with Citrus Quinoa
11	Egg-ocado Toast with Cherry Tomatoes and Feta	Spicy Thai Peanut Veggie Wrap (reduce wrap portion)	Spicy Tamari Trail Mix	Cauliflower Rice with Citrus Shrimp
12	Caprese Avocado Toast with Soft Boiled Egg	Quinoa-Stuffed Baked Salmon	Berry Lavender Greek Yogurt Cups	Spaghetti Squash with Marinara and Turkey Meatballs
13	Savory Spinach and Feta Whole Grain Pancakes	Sweet Potato and Kale Stir-Fry	Classic Chewy Oatmeal Raisin Cookies	Braised Spaghetti Squash with Chermoula and Crumbled Feta
14	Pistachio and Matcha Greek Yogurt Delight	Sun-Dried Tomato and Almond Pesto Zucchini Noodles	Avocado Lime Hummus with Herbed Veggie Sticks	Spicy Shrimp Over Lime Infused Cauliflower Rice

Tips for Success

1. **Balance Your Plate:** Focus on filling half your plate with vegetables, a quarter with lean protein, and the remaining quarter with whole grains or other complex carbs. This balance helps manage blood sugar levels and keeps you satisfied.

2. **Modify Recipes As Needed:** If a recipe or meal idea seems too bland, don't hesitate to modify it. Spices and seasonings like paprika, garlic powder, or cumin can add flavor without extra calories or carbs.

3. **Be Consistent with Portions:** Even as your carb intake lowers, it's crucial to maintain consistent portion sizes to ensure you're receiving enough energy and nutrients. Use measuring cups or a food scale if you're unsure about portion sizes.

4. **Stay Flexible with Meal Timing:** If your schedule changes, it's okay to adjust meal times. What's important is maintaining the overall structure and balance of your meals, not necessarily the clock time they are consumed.

5. **Listen to Your Hunger Cues:** Pay attention to your body's signals. If you're consistently hungry, you may need to slightly increase protein or fiber at your meals, which can provide longer-lasting satiety.

6. **Prepare for Challenges:** The middle weeks can sometimes feel challenging as the novelty wears off and reality sets in. Keep your motivation high by reminding yourself of your progress and the health benefits you're starting to experience.

7. **Stay Connected with Your Support System:** Share your experiences, swap recipes, or discuss challenges with others who are on similar paths. Support can make a significant difference in maintaining motivation.

Continuing with Meal Plan 2, you are likely to start feeling stronger in your ability to control portions and make smart, instinctive choices about food. Let this newfound confidence build as you prepare to take on the final phase of your carb cycling plan. Remember, these steps are not just about reducing carb intake; they're about creating a more mindful and healthier relationship with food. That's something to truly be excited about as you move forward.

4. MEAL PLAN 3: WEEKS 5-6

By now, in Weeks 5-6 of our journey, you're familiar with the rhythm and flow of the carb cycling process. Meal Plan 3 takes you further into a low-carb lifestyle, skillfully refining the tools and habits you've built over the past month. This plan encourages fat burning and helps stabilize blood sugar levels as you become acclimated to reduced carbohydrate intake, enhancing both physical and mental energy.

DAY	BREAKFAST	LUNCH	SNACK	DINNER
1	Classic Avocado and Bacon Omelette	Mediterranean Tuna Lettuce Wraps	Rosemary Almond-Crusted Chicken Breast	Garlic Butter Shrimp with Herbed Cauliflower Rice
2	Zesty Lime and Avocado Omelette	Caesar-Style Kale Salad with Grilled Shrimp	Vanilla Almond Crunch Yogurt	Baked Cod with Mediterranean Tomato Concasse
3	Bacon, Avocado, and Goat Cheese Omelette	Classic Zucchini Noodles with Basil Pesto	Lavender Almond Shortbread	Parmesan & Sage Chicken Cutlets with Roasted Vegetables
4	Smoked Salmon and Spinach Frittata Muffins	Classic Tuna Salad Lettuce Wraps	Maple Cinnamon Seed Crunch	Szechuan Beef and Broccoli Stir-Fry
5	Shiitake Mushroom and Gruyere Egg Muffins	Grilled Chicken Caesar Salad	Spiced Almond Cookies	Baked Cod with Caper and Lemon Butter Sauce
6	Kale and Parmesan Egg Muffins	Classic Zucchini Noodles with Basil Pesto	Classic Almond Flour Cookies	Seared Tuna Caesar Salad
7	Chorizo and Egg White Muffins	Asian Zest Tuna Lettuce Wraps	Savory Rosemary Nut Mix	Lemon-Thyme Chicken with Herb Crust
8	Classic Avocado and Bacon Omelette	Caesar-Style Kale Salad with Grilled Shrimp	Vanilla Almond Crunch Yogurt	Baked Cod with Mediterranean Tomato Concasse
9	Zesty Lime and Avocado Omelette	Avocado Pesto Zucchini Noodles	Lemon-Thyme Chicken with Herb Crust	Parmesan & Sage Chicken Cutlets with Roasted Vegetables

10	Smoked Salmon and Spinach Frittata Muffins	Mediterranean Tuna Lettuce Wraps	Spiced Almond Cookies	Szechuan Beef and Broccoli Stir-Fry
11	Kale and Parmesan Egg Muffins	Grilled Chicken Caesar Salad	Maple Cinnamon Seed Crunch	Rosemary Almond-Crusted Chicken Breast
12	Bacon, Avocado, and Goat Cheese Omelette	Classic Zucchini Noodles with Basil Pesto	Lavender Almond Shortbread	Spicy Lemon Grass Beef with Steamed Vegetables
13	Chorizo and Egg White Muffins	Asian Zest Tuna Lettuce Wraps	Savory Rosemary Nut Mix	Garlic Butter Shrimp with Herbed Cauliflower Rice
14	Shiitake Mushroom and Gruyere Egg Muffins	Mediterranean Tuna Lettuce Wraps	Vanilla Almond Crunch Yogurt	Baked Cod with Caper and Lemon Butter Sauce

Tips for Success

1. **Embrace Variety:** To avoid dietary boredom, particularly in a low-carb phase, explore a variety of spices and seasonings to enhance the flavor without adding extra carbs. Consider incorporating more international dishes that leverage spices creatively.

2. **Maintain Meal Balance:** Even with reduced carbs, ensure your meals are balanced with adequate protein and healthy fats. This balance is crucial for maintaining muscle mass and overall satiety.

3. **Monitor Your Body's Response:** As carbs go lower, some might experience changes in energy or mood. If you feel overly fatigued, consider adjusting your intake slightly. There's room to tweak and adjust based on how you feel.

4. **Hydration is Key:** Lower carb intake might result in less water retention, so increasing your water intake is crucial to maintain hydration, aid digestion, and keep your energy levels stable.

5. **Plan Ahead for Challenges:** Low-carb diets can be challenging to stick to, especially in social settings. Plan ahead by preparing appropriate snacks and meals that you can bring to social gatherings or knowing menu items that fit your dietary needs when dining out.

6. **Keep Connected with Support:** Continue to engage with others who are on the same path. Sharing your experiences can provide new ideas and motivation to stick with your goals.

7. **Reflect on Your Progress:** Take time to appreciate how far you've come. Reflecting on the changes in your body, your attitude towards food, and your overall health can be incredibly motivating as you near the end of this initial structured plan.

Meal Plan 3 is your stepping stone towards mastering a lifestyle with reduced carbohydrates. It's designed not just for weight loss but for a deeper, sustainable integration of healthy eating habits into your life. As you continue to apply these principles, remember that each meal is an opportunity to nourish and celebrate your body's journey towards better health.

CHAPTER 7: HIGH-CARB DAY RECIPES

1. BREAKFAST RECIPES

A burst of morning energy encapsulated in a meal—this is precisely what our high-carb day breakfast recipes promise. We know that mornings can often dictate the rhythm of your entire day. It's not just about filling up but fueling up intelligently with choices that energize, satisfy, and set a positive tone as you step into the daylight hustles or serene beginnings, depending on your schedule.

Imagine this: You're waking to the aroma of oatmeal swirling with fresh berries, their vibrant hues peeking out invitingly. Or perhaps the comfort of whole grain pancakes, slightly crispy on the edges, soft in the center, accompanied by a melody of toppings that add not just flavor but a nutritional punch. These aren't just meals; they're experiences that encourage you to embrace the day's challenges with enthusiasm.

Whether you're an early riser prepping for a day packed with meetings or a stay-at-home parent orchestrating morning routines, these breakfasts are designed to align with those elevated carbohydrate days, providing you with sustained energy. The science behind carb cycling isn't just about reducing or increasing carb intake whimsically. It's about timing and pairing—ensuring your high-carb choices support your body's peak activity times. Breakfast, being your first meal, sets that energetic blueprint for the day.

And while the delicious simplicity of a fruit smoothie bowl or the hearty satisfaction of a well-assembled quinoa black bean salad might feel like indulgences, they're strategically crafted to enhance your metabolic efficiency. These meals are your morning allies, assisting in not just weight management but also in achieving a clarity of mind and a lightness of spirit.

So, let's turn each breakfast into a small celebration of new beginnings. With these recipes, we're not just eating; we are also setting intentions, fueling aspirations, and preparing physically and mentally for the opportunities ahead. The kitchen transforms into a place of preparation and empowerment, where every dish is an affirmation of your health and happiness goals. Let's break the fast with a zeal for life, one high-carb day at a time.

OATMEAL WITH FRESH BERRIES

CLASSIC VANILLA OATMEAL WITH FRESH BERRIES

P.T.: 5 min. | **C.T.:** 10 min.

M. of C.: Stovetop | **SERVES:** 2

INGR: 1 C. rolled oats

- 2 C. water

- Pinch of salt

- 1 tsp vanilla extract

- ½ C. fresh strawberries, hulled and sliced

- ½ C. fresh blueberries

- 1 Tbls honey

- 2 Tbls flaxseed meal

- ¼ C. almond milk

PROC: Combine rolled oats, water, and a pinch of salt in a saucepan and bring to a boil over medium-high heat

- Reduce heat and simmer, stirring occasionally, until oats are tender and have absorbed most of the water, about 5 to 7 min.

- Remove from heat, stir in vanilla extract, flaxseed meal, and almond milk

- Serve oats topped with fresh strawberries, blueberries, and a drizzle of honey

TIPS: Add a sprinkle of cinnamon for a warming spice flavor - Use agave syrup as a vegan alternative to honey if desired

N.V.: Calories: 295, Fat: 7g, Carbs: 53g, Protein: 8g, Sugar: 15g

SPIRITED RASPBERRY CHIA OATMEAL

P.T.: 8 min. | **C.T.:** 3 hr. chilling
M. of C.: No Cooking | **SERVES:** 1
INGR: ½ C. rolled oats

- ¾ C. coconut milk
- 1 Tbls chia seeds
- 1 tsp lemon zest
- ½ C. fresh raspberries
- 1 Tbls maple syrup
- 1 Tbls shredded unsweetened coconut

PROC: In a jar, mix rolled oats, coconut milk, chia seeds, and lemon zest

- Stir well until combined and let sit for 5 min.
- Add fresh raspberries and gently fold them into the mixture
- Cover the jar and refrigerate for at least 3 hr. or overnight
- Before serving, top with maple syrup and shredded coconut

TIPS: Try using different berries like blueberries or blackberries for variety - To enhance flavor, add a splash of vanilla extract
N.V.: Calories: 320, Fat: 15g, Carbs: 44g, Protein: 8g, Sugar: 12g

GOLDEN TURMERIC OATMEAL

P.T.: 7 min. | **C.T.:** 15 min.
M. of C.: Stovetop | **SERVES:** 2
INGR: 1 C. steel-cut oats

- 2½ C. water
- 1 C. light coconut milk
- 1 tsp turmeric powder
- Pinch of black pepper
- 1 Tbls golden raisins
- 1 small apple, diced
- 1 Tbls crushed almonds

PROC: In a pot, mix steel-cut oats, water, coconut milk, turmeric powder, and a pinch of black pepper

- Bring to a boil, then reduce heat to low and simmer, stirring occasionally, until oats are tender and creamy, about 15 min.
- Stir in golden raisins and diced apple during the last 3 min. of cooking
- Serve garnished with crushed almonds

TIPS: Experiment with adding a dash of cinnamon or nutmeg for extra spice - Enhance sweetness with a spoon of honey if desired
N.V.: Calories: 275, Fat: 9g, Carbs: 44g, Protein: 6g, Sugar: 10g

BERRY ALMOND OVERNIGHT OATS

P.T.: 10 min. | **C.T.:** 8 hr. chilling
M. of C.: No Cooking | **SERVES:** 2
INGR: 1 C. rolled oats

- 1½ C. almond milk
- 1 Tbls almond butter
- 2 tsp chia seeds
- ¼ C. fresh mixed berries
- 2 tsp honey
- 1 Tbls sliced almonds
- ½ tsp ground cinnamon

PROC: In a mixing bowl, whisk together almond milk, almond butter, chia seeds, and ground cinnamon

- Add rolled oats to the mixture and stir until well coated
- Divide the mixture between two jars
- Top each jar with mixed berries and drizzle with honey
- Seal the jars and refrigerate overnight
- Serve chilled, garnished with sliced almonds

TIPS: Stir before eating to redistribute flavors and textures - For a protein boost, add a scoop of your favorite vanilla or unflavored protein powder
N.V.: Calories: 310, Fat: 12g, Carbs: 46g, Protein: 10g, Sugar: 12g

WHOLE GRAIN PANCAKES

BLUEBERRY BUCKWHEAT PANCAKES

P.T.: 15 min | **C.T.:** 10 min

M. of C.: Pan Frying | **SERVES:** 4

INGR: 1 C. buckwheat flour

- 1 C. all-purpose flour

- 2 Tbls granulated sugar

- 1 Tbls baking powder

- ½ tsp salt

- 2 large eggs, beaten

- 1¾ C. milk

- ¼ C. unsalted butter, melted

- 1 tsp vanilla extract

- 1 C. fresh blueberries

PROC: In a large bowl, whisk together buckwheat flour, all-purpose flour, sugar, baking powder, and salt

- In another bowl, combine beaten eggs, milk, melted butter, and vanilla extract

- Pour the wet ingredients into the dry ingredients and mix until just combined, careful not to overmix

- Gently fold in fresh blueberries

- Heat a non-stick skillet over medium heat and grease lightly

- Pour ¼ C. of batter for each pancake and cook until bubbles form on the surface and edges start to look set, about 2-3 min.; flip and cook until golden brown, about 2 min. more

TIPS: Avoid overmixing the batter to keep pancakes fluffy - Serve with real maple syrup or a dollop of Greek yogurt to boost protein

N.V.: Calories: 210, Fat: 7g, Carbs: 32g, Protein: 6g, Sugar: 8g

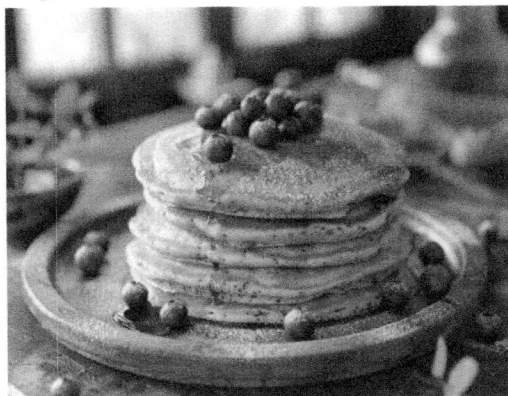

CINNAMON SWIRL WHOLE GRAIN PANCAKES

P.T.: 20 min | **C.T.:** 15 min

M. of C.: Pan Frying | **SERVES:** 6

INGR: 2 C. whole wheat flour

- 1 Tbls baking powder

- ½ tsp salt

- 1 Tbls ground cinnamon

- 2 Tbls brown sugar

- 2 large eggs

- 1½ C. buttermilk

- 4 Tbls unsalted butter, melted

- 1 tsp vanilla extract

- ¼ C. cinnamon sugar for swirling

PROC: Combine whole wheat flour, baking powder, salt, ground cinnamon, and brown sugar in a large mixing bowl

- In a separate bowl, whisk together eggs, buttermilk, melted butter, and vanilla extract

- Gradually mix the wet ingredients into the dry ingredients until just combined

- Preheat a griddle over medium heat and grease lightly

- Pour about ¼ C. batter per pancake onto the griddle

- Sprinkle approximately 1 tsp of cinnamon sugar on top and use a knife to swirl it into the batter

- Cook until bubbles form on the surface, then flip and cook until golden brown, about 3-4 min. total

TIPS: Use a squeeze bottle to create finer cinnamon swirls in the batter - Pair these pancakes with sliced apples for added freshness and crunch - Mix some cream cheese with a little honey and spread on top for a creamy finish

N.V.: Calories: 255, Fat: 11g, Carbs: 34g, Protein: 7g, Sugar: 10g

SAVORY SPINACH AND FETA WHOLE GRAIN PANCAKES

P.T.: 20 min | **C.T.:** 15 min
M. of C.: Pan Frying | **SERVES:** 4
INGR: 1½ C. whole wheat flour

- 1 Tbls baking powder

- ½ tsp salt

- 1 Tbls sugar

- 2 Tbls olive oil

- 1 C. milk

- 2 eggs

- ½ C. feta cheese, crumbled

- 1 C. spinach, finely chopped

- 1 small onion, finely diced

- 2 cloves garlic, minced

PROC: Stir together whole wheat flour, baking powder, salt, and sugar in a large bowl

- In another bowl, whisk eggs, milk, and olive oil until well combined

- Add the wet ingredients to the dry ingredients and stir until just mixed

- Fold in crumbled feta, finely chopped spinach, diced onion, and minced garlic

- Heat a non-stick pan over medium heat and lightly oil the surface

- Pour about ¼ C. of batter for each pancake, cooking until the edges are dry and bubbles begin to appear, about 2-3 min.; flip and cook until browned on the other side, about 2 min. more

TIPS: Serve with a dollop of yogurt and a squeeze of lemon for extra zest - These pancakes can be made ahead and reheated for a quick savory breakfast or dinner side- Add a dash of nutmeg to the batter to enhance the flavors of spinach and feta

N.V.: Calories: 280, Fat: 15g, Carbs: 28g, Protein: 10g, Sugar: 4g

FRUIT SMOOTHIE BOWL

TROPICAL MANGO-PAPAYA SMOOTHIE BOWL

P.T.: 15 min | **C.T.:** 0 min
M. of C.: No Cooking | **SERVES:** 2
INGR: 1 C. mango, cubed

- 1 C. papaya, cubed

- 1 banana

- 1/2 C. orange juice

- 1/2 C. Greek yogurt

- 2 Tbls honey

- 1/4 C. granola

- 1 Tbls chia seeds

- 1 Tbls coconut flakes

- 1/4 C. kiwi, sliced

PROC: Blend mango, papaya, banana, orange juice, and Greek yogurt until smooth

- Pour into bowls

- Top with granola, chia seeds, coconut flakes, and kiwi slices

TIPS: Serve immediately for best texture and flavor - Customize toppings with other seasonal fruits or nuts for variety - Use a high-speed blender for a creamier texture

N.V.: Calories: 350, Fat: 5g, Carbs: 70g, Protein: 9g, Sugar: 48g

BERRY ALMOND SMOOTHIE BOWL

P.T.: 10 min | **C.T.:** 0 min

M. of C.: No Cooking | **SERVES:** 1

INGR: 1 C. frozen mixed berries

- 1/2 C. Greek yogurt

- 1/4 C. almond milk

- 1 Tbls almond butter

- 1/2 banana

- 2 Tbls sliced almonds

- 1 Tbls hemp seeds

- 1 Tsp honey

PROC: Combine frozen berries, Greek yogurt, almond milk, almond butter, and banana in a blender and blend until smooth

- Pour mixture into a bowl

- Garnish with sliced almonds, hemp seeds, and a drizzle of honey

TIPS: Add a scoop of protein powder for an extra protein boost - Substitute honey with maple syrup if desired for a different sweetness - Ensure to use unsweetened almond milk to keep sugar content in control

N.V.: Calories: 325, Fat: 15g, Carbs: 40g, Protein: 12g, Sugar: 25g

GREEN KIWI SMOOTHIE BOWL

P.T.: 12 min | **C.T.:** 0 min

M. of C.: No Cooking | **SERVES:** 2

INGR: 2 ripe kiwis, peeled and sliced

- 1/2 avocado

- 1/2 C. spinach leaves

- 1/2 C. coconut water

- 1/2 banana

- 2 Tbls pumpkin seeds

- 1 Tbls flax seeds

- 1/4 C. blueberries

- 1 Tbls honey

PROC: Blend kiwis, avocado, spinach, coconut water, and banana until smooth

- Transfer to bowls

- Sprinkle pumpkin seeds, flax seeds, and blueberries on top

- Drizzle with honey

TIPS: Freeze the banana before blending for a thicker texture - Adjust sweetness by varying the amount of honey according to taste - Incorporate a scoop of green superfood powder for added nutrients

N.V.: Calories: 290, Fat: 10g, Carbs: 48g, Protein: 6g, Sugar: 32g

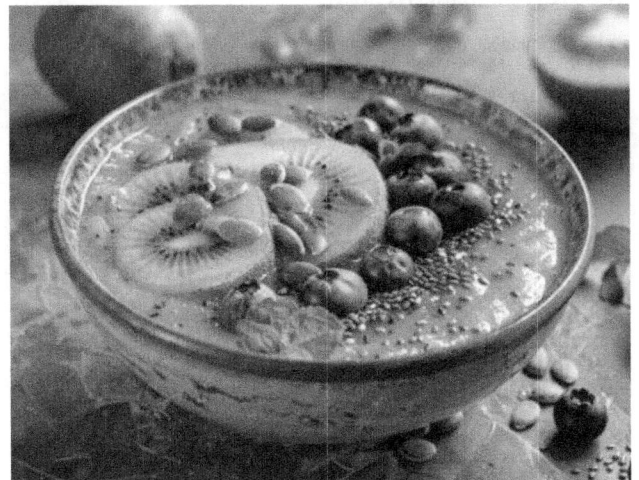

2. LUNCH RECIPES

As we stroll through our culinary journey tailored for high-carb days, it becomes clear how these meals not only offer comfort and satisfaction but dive deeper into supporting vigorous energy levels, necessary for those more active days. Particularly at lunch, a vital meal that sets the tone for the afternoon's pace, the perfect balance of intricate carbs offers not just nourishment but a much-needed zest to push through the latter part of the day.

Imagine sitting down to a spread that blends both flavor and function. High-carb doesn't simply mean indulgent pastas and bread—heavenly as they are! It extends to foods rich in fiber, essential vitamins, and minerals, which release energy steadily. This ensures you don't face that all-too-familiar mid-afternoon slump. The creations you'll discover here—think quinoa and black bean salad brimming with colorful veggies, or a lively chicken and brown rice stir-fry—are crafted to be as delightful to palette as they are beneficial for your body.

Each ingredient is selected to fortify your meal with an energizing boost. Quinoa, for instance, is not just a carb; it's a complete protein, rich in fiber and amino acids, which supports muscle repair and growth—ideal for recovery if your morning involved intense physical activity. The black beans complement this with their high protein content and heart-healthy fiber, making each forkful a step towards sustained energy levels.

These recipes also honor our commitment to meals that cater to the whole family. Easy to prepare and even easier to love, they fit seamlessly into your dynamic lifestyle without compromising on health or taste. As you whisk through these recipes, you'll find each dish is not just a meal but a building block to a lifelong habit of smart, balanced eating.

Steering through these high-carb treasures, you'll feel equipped—ready to craft lunches that are as nourishing as they are energizing. They're more than just recipes; they're your secret weapon for maintaining momentum, both physically and mentally, throughout your bustling days.

QUINOA AND BLACK BEAN SALAD

TROPICAL QUINOA AND BLACK BEAN SALAD

P.T.: 20 min | **C.T.:** 25 min

M. of C.: Boiling and Mixing | **SERVES:** 4

INGR: 1 C. quinoa, rinsed

- 2 C. water

- 1 can (15 oz.) black beans, drained and rinsed

- 1 mango, peeled and diced

- 1 red bell pepper, diced

- 1 avocado, peeled, pitted, and chopped

- 1/4 C. fresh cilantro, chopped

- Juice of 2 limes

- 2 Tbls extra virgin olive oil

- 1 tsp cumin

- Salt and pepper to taste

PROC: Combine water and quinoa in a saucepan and bring to a boil

- Reduce heat to low, cover, and simmer until quinoa is tender and water has been absorbed, about 15 min

- Fluff quinoa with a fork and allow to cool slightly

- In a large bowl, combine cooled quinoa, black beans, mango, red bell pepper, and avocado

- In a small bowl, whisk together lime juice, olive oil, cumin, salt, and pepper

- Pour dressing over the salad and toss gently to combine

- Garnish with fresh cilantro

TIPS: Serve chilled or at room temperature for best flavor - Adding a pinch of chili flakes can give a pleasant heat to the dish - If mango is not in season, peaches make an excellent substitute

N.V.: Calories: 310, Fat: 10g, Carbs: 49g, Protein: 9g, Sugar: 6g

MEDITERRANEAN QUINOA AND BLACK BEAN SALAD

P.T.: 15 min | **C.T.:** 0 min

M. of C.: Mixing | **SERVES:** 4

INGR: 1 C. cooked quinoa, cooled

- 1 can (15 oz.) black beans, drained and rinsed

- 1/2 C. Kalamata olives, pitted and sliced

- 1/2 C. feta cheese, crumbled

- 1 cucumber, diced

- 1/2 red onion, finely chopped

- 1/4 C. sun-dried tomatoes, chopped

- 2 Tbls olive oil

- 3 Tbls red wine vinegar

- 1 Tbls dried oregano

- Salt and pepper to taste

PROC: In a large bowl, mix together quinoa, black beans, olives, feta cheese, cucumber, red onion, and sun-dried tomatoes

- In a small bowl, combine olive oil, red wine vinegar, oregano, salt, and pepper to create the dressing

- Pour dressing over the salad ingredients and toss to coat evenly

TIPS: This salad can be stored in the refrigerator for up to three days, making it a great make-ahead meal option - Try adding a handful of fresh arugula or spinach for extra greens - Drizzle with a bit of lemon juice just before serving for added zest

N.V.: Calories: 290, Fat: 15g, Carbs: 33g, Protein: 9g, Sugar: 5g

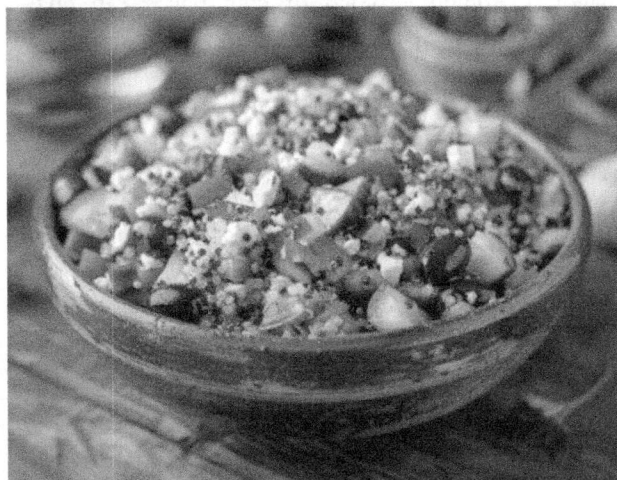

CURRY QUINOA AND BLACK BEAN SALAD

P.T.: 15 min | **C.T.:** 0 min

M. of C.: Mixing | **SERVES:** 4

INGR: 1 C. cooked quinoa, cooled

- 1 can (15 oz.) black beans, rinsed and drained

- 1 small red bell pepper, diced

- 1 small yellow bell pepper, diced

- 1/2 C. raisins

- 1/4 C. slivered almonds

- 1/4 C. fresh parsley, chopped

- 2 Tbls curry powder

- 1 Tbls honey

- Juice of 1 lemon

- 3 Tbls olive oil

- Salt to taste

PROC: In a large mixing bowl, combine quinoa, black beans, red and yellow bell peppers, raisins, almonds, and parsley

- In a separate small bowl, whisk together curry powder, honey, lemon juice, olive oil, and salt to make the dressing

- Drizzle the dressing over the quinoa mixture and toss until everything is well-coated

TIPS: Consider toasting the almonds before adding them to the salad for a deeper flavor - Serve this salad with a dollop of Greek yogurt on top for a creamy texture and a balance to the spices - Leftovers make excellent stuffed fillings for bell peppers or tomatoes

N.V.: Calories: 275, Fat: 8g, Carbs: 44g, Protein: 8g, Sugar: 10g

CHICKEN AND BROWN RICE STIR-FRY

THAI BASIL CHICKEN AND BROWN RICE STIR-FRY

P.T.: 15 min | **C.T.:** 20 min

M. of C.: Stovetop | **SERVES:** 4

INGR: 2 C. brown rice, uncooked

- 1 lb. chicken breast, thinly sliced

- 1 red bell pepper, julienned

- 1 C. fresh Thai basil leaves

- 2 Tbls soy sauce

- 1 Tbls fish sauce

- 1 Tbls oyster sauce

- 2 tsp brown sugar

- 3 cloves garlic, minced

- 2 Tbls vegetable oil

- 1/2 tsp crushed red pepper flakes

- 1/4 C. water

PROC: Cook brown rice according to package instructions and set aside

- Heat oil in a large skillet over medium-high heat

- Add garlic and red pepper flakes, sauté until fragrant

- Add chicken and cook until browned

- Add bell pepper and stir-fry for 2-3 minutes

- Combine soy sauce, fish sauce, oyster sauce, brown sugar, and water in a bowl, stir well

- Pour the sauce mixture into the skillet, bring to a boil, and reduce to simmer for 5 min

- Stir in Thai basil leaves just before serving over brown rice

TIPS: Opt to garnish with additional basil leaves for enhanced flavor and presentation - Use low-sodium soy sauce to control salt intake - Squeeze a lime wedge over the dish before eating for an added zesty flavor

N.V.: Calories: 350, Fat: 8g, Carbs: 48g, Protein: 28g, Sugar: 3g

MANGO AND CHICKEN BROWN RICE PILAF

P.T.: 10 min | **C.T.:** 25 min

M. of C.: Stovetop | **SERVES:** 4

INGR: 1 C. brown rice

- 1 lb. chicken thighs, boneless and skinless, cubed

- 1 ripe mango, cubed

- 1 medium onion, chopped

- 1 red bell pepper, diced

- 3 Tbls olive oil

- 1 tsp ground turmeric

- 1 tsp cumin seeds

- 1/2 C. chicken broth

- Salt and pepper to taste

- Fresh cilantro, chopped for garnish

PROC: Cook brown rice as per package instructions

- Heat olive oil in a skillet over medium heat, add cumin seeds and turmeric, toast briefly

- Add onions and bell pepper, sauté until onions are translucent

- Add chicken, season with salt and pepper, and brown on all sides

- Add cooked rice, mango, and chicken broth to the skillet, stir well, and cover to simmer for 10 min

- Garnish with cilantro before serving

TIPS: Utilize ripe mangos for a natural sweetness that complements the spices - Can substitute cilantro with parsley if preferred - Adding a pinch of cinnamon can offer a warm spice undertone

N.V.: Calories: 390, Fat: 14g, Carbs: 45g, Protein: 25g, Sugar: 8g

CHICKEN SHAWARMA BROWN RICE BOWL

P.T.: 20 min | **C.T.:** 30 min
M. of C.: Stovetop | **SERVES:** 4
INGR: 2 C. brown rice

- 1 lb. chicken breast, thinly sliced
- 1 Tbls ground coriander
- 1 Tbls ground cumin
- 1 tsp smoked paprika
- 1/2 tsp cayenne pepper
- 3 garlic cloves, minced
- Juice of 1 lemon
- 3 Tbls olive oil
- 1 cucumber, diced
- 2 tomatoes, diced
- 1/2 red onion, thinly sliced
- Greek yogurt, for serving
- Fresh mint leaves, for garnish

PROC: Cook brown rice according to package instructions

- In a bowl, mix lemon juice, 2 Tbls olive oil, coriander, cumin, paprika, cayenne, and minced garlic to create marinade

- Toss chicken in marinade and let sit for at least 10 min

- Heat remaining olive oil in a skillet over medium heat and cook chicken until browned

- Assemble rice bowls with cooked rice, cooked chicken, cucumber, tomatoes, and red onion

- Top with a dollop of Greek yogurt and garnish with mint leaves

TIPS: Marinate chicken overnight for deeper flavor infusion - Serve with a side of tahini sauce for added creaminess and tang - Squeeze additional lemon over the bowl for a fresh lift

N.V.: Calories: 410, Fat: 12g, Carbs: 55g, Protein: 27g, Sugar: 5g

SWEET POTATO AND LENTIL SOUP

CURRIED SWEET POTATO AND LENTIL SOUP

P.T.: 15 min. | **C.T.:** 40 min.
M. of C.: Stovetop | **SERVES:** 4
INGR: 2 Tbls coconut oil

- 1 large onion, diced
- 2 cloves garlic, minced
- 1 Tbls fresh ginger, grated
- 1 Tbls curry powder
- 4 C. vegetable broth
- 2 large sweet potatoes, peeled and cubed
- 1 C. red lentils
- 1 tsp salt
- 1/2 tsp ground black pepper
- 1 can (14 oz.) coconut milk
- Fresh cilantro, chopped for garnish

PROC: Heat coconut oil in a large pot over medium heat

- Add onion, garlic, and ginger; cook until onion is translucent

- Stir in curry powder and cook for 1 min

- Add vegetable broth, sweet potatoes, and lentils; bring to a boil

- Reduce heat and simmer until sweet potatoes and lentils are tender, about 30 min

- Stir in coconut milk and season with salt and pepper; cook for additional 10 min

- Serve garnished with cilantro

TIPS: Add a squeeze of lime juice for added zest - Serve with naan bread for dipping - Can be stored in the refrigerator for up to 3 days or frozen for longer storage

N.V.: Calories: 376, Fat: 13g, Carbs: 54g, Protein: 13g, Sugar: 7g

SWEET POTATO AND LENTIL SOUP WITH SMOKY PAPRIKA

P.T.: 20 min. | **C.T.:** 45 min.

M. of C.: Stovetop | **SERVES:** 6

INGR: 1 Tbls olive oil

- 1 medium red onion, chopped

- 2 Tbls smoked paprika

- 1 Tbls cumin seeds

- 3 medium sweet potatoes, peeled and diced

- 1 1/2 C. brown lentils

- 6 C. chicken or vegetable stock

- 2 tsp apple cider vinegar

- Salt and pepper to taste

- Chopped scallions for garnish

PROC: Heat olive oil in a large saucepan over medium heat

- Add red onion and sauté until soft

- Add smoked paprika and cumin seeds, toast for 2 min

- Add sweet potatoes, lentils, and stock; bring to a boil

- Lower the heat and simmer until lentils are cooked and sweet potatoes are tender, about 35 min

- Stir in apple cider vinegar, season with salt and pepper

- Serve hot, garnished with scallions

TIPS: Try adding a dollop of sour cream on top for creaminess - This recipe pairs well with a crispy green salad - Leftovers make a robust base for a shepherd's pie filling

N.V.: Calories: 330, Fat: 5g, Carbs: 53g, Protein: 18g, Sugar: 9g

THAI-INSPIRED SWEET POTATO AND LENTIL SOUP

P.T.: 20 min. | **C.T.:** 50 min.

M. of C.: Stovetop | **SERVES:** 4

INGR: 1 Tbls sesame oil

- 1 leek, white and light green parts finely sliced

- 1 Tbls Thai red curry paste

- 4 C. vegetable stock

- 2 medium sweet potatoes, peeled and cubed

- 1 C. green lentils

- 1 fl. oz. fish sauce

- 1 can (14 oz.) coconut milk

- Chopped basil and mint for garnish

PROC: Heat sesame oil in a soup pot over medium flame

- Add leek and sauté until tender

- Stir in Thai red curry paste and cook for 2 min

- Pour in vegetable stock and bring to a simmer

- Add sweet potatoes and lentils; cover and simmer until tender, about 40 min

- Add fish sauce and coconut milk, heat through

- Serve hot, garnished with fresh basil and mint leaves

TIPS: Incorporate a few drops of lime juice for a refreshing twist - Perfect with steamed jasmine rice - Consider adding diced tofu for extra protein

N.V.: Calories: 390, Fat: 15g, Carbs: 50g, Protein: 16g, Sugar: 8g

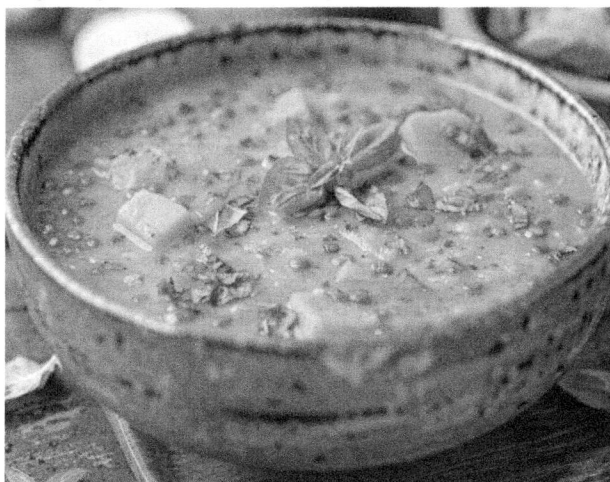

3. DINNER RECIPES

As the sun begins to set and the busy whirl of daytime activities winds down, dinner stands as a pivotal moment in our carb cycling journey—especially on our high-carb days. For many, evenings are a gathering time; a chance to come together with loved ones around the dinner table. This is where our high-carb dinner recipes step in, crafted to encourage this togetherness, while also fueling your body with the right energy sources to capitalize on tomorrow's activities.

In this chapter, we explore a variety of dinner recipes that blend traditional comfort with nutritional ingenuity. Each recipe is thoughtfully designed to make your high-carb days both delightful and effective for your health goals. We move beyond the usual plate of pasta, introducing you to meals like a heart-warming Whole Wheat Pasta Primavera, a hearty baked salmon sided with quinoa, and a veggie-packed stir-fry that bursts with both color and flavor.

These recipes keep multiple factors in mind—ease of preparation after a long day, the nutritional balance needed to keep your energy levels consistent, and of course, the pleasure of good taste. What's more, these meals are crafted to appeal to all members of the family, ensuring that your journey towards health and wellness is a shared and enjoyable experience. After all, sticking to a plan is easier when it's embraced as a collective effort.

Imagine this: A dinner of Baked Salmon with Quinoa, rich in omega-3 fatty acids from the salmon and complete proteins from the quinoa, powers up your body's recovery processes through the night. Meanwhile, the fibrous quinoa assists in those high-carb benefits without letting your blood sugar levels spike and crash. It's not just a dish; it's a strategic inclusion to your diet plan that is as delicious as it is nutritious.

As we delve into these recipes, consider how they serve not just your body's needs, but also your soul's craving for community and connection at the dinner table. Here's to dinners that are more than just eating: they're about enriching your body and your bonds.

WHOLE WHEAT PASTA PRIMAVERA

SPRING VEGETABLE WHOLE WHEAT PASTA PRIMAVERA

P.T.: 20 min | **C.T.:** 15 min

M. of C.: Boiling and Sautéing | **SERVES:** 4

INGR: 350g whole wheat pasta

- 1 C. fresh asparagus, trimmed and cut into 1-inch pieces

- 1 C. sugar snap peas, trimmed

- 1 medium carrot, julienned

- 1 small zucchini, sliced

- 1 yellow bell pepper, sliced

- 4 Tbls extra virgin olive oil

- 2 cloves garlic, minced

- 1 tsp dried Italian seasoning

- ½ C. cherry tomatoes, halved

- ¼ C. freshly grated Parmesan cheese

- Salt and black pepper to taste

PROC: Cook pasta in boiling water until al dente, drain and set aside

- In a large skillet, heat olive oil over medium heat and sauté garlic, asparagus, snap peas, carrot, zucchini, and bell pepper until tender

- Stir in the cooked pasta, Italian seasoning, cherry tomatoes, and season with salt and black pepper

- Sprinkle Parmesan over the top and serve

TIPS: Serve with a squeeze of fresh lemon juice for additional zest - Pair with a light Chardonnay to complement the fresh flavors

N.V.: Calories: 310, Fat: 14g, Carbs: 38g, Protein: 10g, Sugar: 5g

MEDITERRANEAN WHOLE WHEAT PASTA PRIMAVERA

P.T.: 25 min | **C.T.:** 20 min

M. of C.: Boiling and Sautéing | **SERVES:** 4

INGR: 350g whole wheat spaghetti

- 1 C. artichoke hearts, quartered

- 1 red onion, thinly sliced

- 1 C. roasted red peppers, sliced

- 2 Tbls capers

- 3 Tbls olive oil

- 2 Tbls balsamic vinegar

- 1 tsp dried oregano

- ½ C. black olives, pitted and halved

- ½ C. feta cheese, crumbled

- Fresh basil leaves for garnish

PROC: Cook spaghetti according to package instructions until al dente, drain and set aside

- In a large skillet, heat olive oil and sauté onion, roasted red peppers, and artichoke hearts until softened

- Add capers, balsamic vinegar, and oregano, cook for an additional 5 min

- Combine the vegetable mix with cooked spaghetti, black olives, and crumble feta over the top

- Garnish with fresh basil before serving

TIPS: Add crushed red pepper flakes for a spicy kick - Enjoy this dish chilled during warmer weather as a pasta salad

N.V.: Calories: 365, Fat: 18g, Carbs: 42g, Protein: 12g, Sugar: 4g

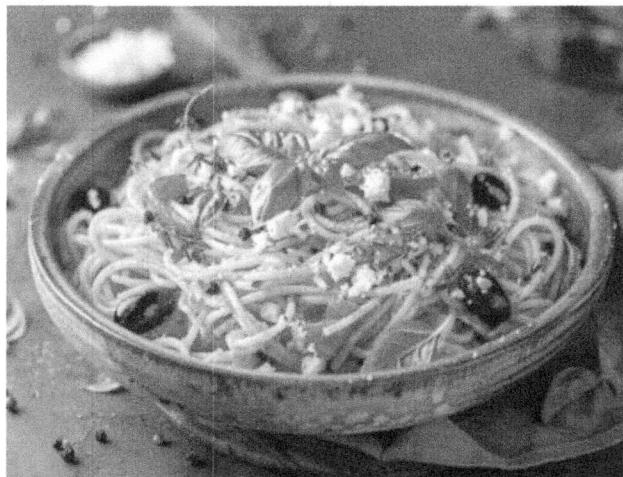

LEMON GARLIC SHRIMP AND WHOLE WHEAT PASTA PRIMAVERA

P.T.: 15 min | **C.T.:** 10 min

M. of C.: Boiling and Sautéing | **SERVES:** 4

INGR: 350g whole wheat linguine

- 2 Tbls olive oil

- 1 lb. shrimp, peeled and deveined

- 3 garlic cloves, minced

- 1 lemon, zest and juice

- 1 C. cherry tomatoes, halved

- 1 C. arugula

- 1 tsp red chili flakes

- Salt and black pepper to taste

- Fresh parsley, chopped for garnish

PROC: Boil linguine until al dente, drain and set aside

- In a skillet, heat olive oil over medium-high heat, add garlic and shrimp, cook until shrimp are pink and cooked through

- Stir in cherry tomatoes and cook until they begin to soften

- Add lemon zest, lemon juice, and red chili flakes to the skillet, combine well

- Toss the cooked pasta with the shrimp mixture, add arugula, and season with salt and pepper

- Garnish with fresh parsley before serving

TIPS: Serve immediately to enjoy the freshness of the arugula and lemon - Use high-quality extra virgin olive oil for the best flavor

N.V.: Calories: 330, Fat: 12g, Carbs: 35g, Protein: 25g, Sugar: 3g

BAKED SALMON WITH QUINOA

HERBED BAKED SALMON WITH CITRUS QUINOA

P.T.: 15 min. | **C.T.:** 20 min.

M. of C.: Baking | **SERVES:** 4

INGR: 4 salmon fillets (6 oz. each)

- 2 Tbls extra virgin olive oil

- 1 Tbls fresh lemon juice

- 2 garlic cloves, minced

- 1 tsp dried dill

- 1 tsp dried parsley

- Salt and pepper to taste

- 1 C. quinoa

- 2 C. water

- Zest of one orange

- Juice of one orange

- 1 Tbls fresh chives, chopped

PROC: Preheat oven to 375°F (190°C)

- In a bowl, mix olive oil, lemon juice, minced garlic, dill, parsley, salt, and pepper

- Brush the salmon fillets with the marinade and let rest for 10 min.

- Meanwhile, rinse quinoa under cold water until water runs clear

- In a saucepan, bring 2 C. water to a boil, add quinoa, reduce heat to low, cover, and simmer for 15 min. until water is absorbed

- Remove from heat and let sit covered for 5 min.

- Fluff quinoa with a fork and mix in orange zest, orange juice, and chives

- Place marinated salmon on a baking sheet lined with parchment paper

- Bake in preheated oven for 20 min. or until salmon flakes easily with a fork

- Serve the baked salmon over citrus quinoa

TIPS: Add a sprig of fresh dill on top of the salmon before serving for enhanced flavor and presentation - Combine leftover citrus quinoa with mixed greens for a refreshing salad the next day

N.V.: Calories: 400, Fat: 15g, Carbs: 30g, Protein: 35g, Sugar: 3g

QUINOA-STUFFED BAKED SALMON

P.T.: 20 min. | **C.T.:** 25 min.

M. of C.: Baking | **SERVES:** 4

INGR: 4 salmon fillets (6 oz. each)

- 1 C. cooked quinoa

- 1/2 C. spinach, finely chopped

- 1/4 C. feta cheese, crumbled

- 1/4 C. sun-dried tomatoes, chopped

- 1 Tbls olive oil

- 2 tsp lemon zest

- Salt and pepper to taste

- 1 Tbls fresh basil, chopped

PROC: Preheat oven to 375°F (190°C)

- Combine cooked quinoa, spinach, feta cheese, sun-dried tomatoes, olive oil, lemon zest, salt, and pepper in a bowl

- Cut a slit horizontally across each salmon fillet to create a pocket

- Stuff the quinoa mixture into the pockets of the salmon fillets

- Place stuffed fillets on a greased baking tray

- Bake for 25 min. until salmon is cooked through and flakes easily

- Garnish with fresh basil before serving

TIPS: Serve with a wedge of lemon for extra tanginess

- This dish can be paired with a light Chardonnay to complement the feta and sun-dried tomatoes

N.V.: Calories: 420, Fat: 17g, Carbs: 28g, Protein: 38g, Sugar: 3g

SALMON QUINOA PILAF WITH ASPARAGUS

P.T.: 25 min. | **C.T.:** 15 min.

M. of C.: Sauteing and Baking | **SERVES:** 4

INGR: 2 Tbls butter

- 1 small onion, finely diced

- 1 garlic clove, minced

- 1 C. quinoa

- 2 C. fish stock

- 4 salmon fillets (6 oz. each)

- 1/2 lb. asparagus, trimmed and cut into 1-inch pieces

- Salt and pepper to taste

- Lemon wedges for serving

PROC: Preheat oven to 375°F (190°C)

- Melt butter in a skillet over medium heat

- Add onion and garlic, sauté until translucent

- Add quinoa and toast for 2 min., stirring frequently

- Pour in fish stock, bring to a boil, then reduce heat and simmer uncovered for 10 min.

- Arrange salmon fillets on top of the quinoa

- Scatter asparagus around salmon

- Season with salt and pepper

- Transfer skillet to oven and bake for 15 min., or until salmon is cooked and quinoa is tender

- Serve with lemon wedges

TIPS: A sprinkle of fresh parsley enhances the freshness of the dish - For a crispier texture, broil the salmon in the last 2 min. of cooking

N.V.: Calories: 390, Fat: 14g, Carbs: 34g, Protein: 32g, Sugar: 4g

VEGGIE-PACKED STIR-FRY

COLORFUL VEGGIE STIR-FRY WITH TOFU AND CASHEWS

P.T.: 15 min | **C.T.:** 10 min

M. of C.: Stir-Frying | **SERVES:** 4

INGR: 200g firm tofu, cubed

- 1 Tbls sesame oil

- 2 C. broccoli florets

- 1 C. sliced red bell pepper

- 1 C. snow peas

- 1 C. sliced carrots

- ½ C. cashews, toasted

- 2 Tbls soy sauce

- 1 Tbls hoisin sauce

- 1 tsp grated ginger

- 2 cloves garlic, minced

- 1 Tbls cornstarch mixed with 2 Tbls water

PROC: Heat sesame oil in a large wok over medium-high heat

- Add tofu cubes and stir-fry until golden brown, remove and set aside

- In the same wok, add broccoli, red bell pepper, snow peas, and carrots, stir-fry for about 5 min until veggies are just tender

- Return tofu to the wok, add cashews, soy sauce, hoisin sauce, ginger, and garlic, stir well to combine

- Stir in cornstarch mixture and cook for another 2 min until sauce thickens

TIPS: Add a splash of lime juice for an extra zesty flavor - Serve over a bed of brown rice or quinoa to make it a complete meal

N.V.: Calories: 285, Fat: 15g, Carbs: 24g, Protein: 15g, Sugar: 7g

MEDITERRANEAN VEGGIE AND CHICKPEA SAUTÉ

P.T.: 10 min | **C.T.:** 12 min
M. of C.: Sautéing | **SERVES:** 3
INGR: 1 C. cooked chickpeas

- 1 Tbls olive oil

- ½ C. diced onions

- 2 cloves garlic, minced

- 1 C. diced zucchini

- 1 C. chopped spinach

- ½ C. cherry tomatoes, halved

- ¼ C. Kalamata olives, pitted and sliced

- 1 tsp dried oregano

- Salt and pepper to taste

- Crumbled feta cheese for garnish

PROC: Heat olive oil in a skillet over medium heat

- Sauté onions and garlic until they become translucent, about 3 min

- Add zucchini, chickpeas, and cook for another 5 min until zucchini is soft

- Stir in spinach, cherry tomatoes, olives, oregano, salt, and pepper, cook for additional 4 min until spinach is wilted

- Garnish with feta cheese before serving

TIPS: Sprinkle some lemon zest for a fresh taste - Serve with a slice of whole-grain bread for a heartier meal

N.V.: Calories: 240, Fat: 9g, Carbs: 29g, Protein: 9g, Sugar: 5g

SWEET POTATO AND KALE STIR-FRY

P.T.: 10 min | **C.T.:** 8 min
M. of C.: Stir-Frying | **SERVES:** 2
INGR: 1 large sweet potato, peeled and cut into small cubes

- 1 Tbls coconut oil

- 2 C. kale, chopped

- ½ red onion, sliced

- 2 tsp soy sauce

- 1 tsp maple syrup

- 1 tsp apple cider vinegar

- 1 tsp smoked paprika

- Salt and pepper to taste

- Toasted sesame seeds for garnish

PROC: Heat coconut oil in a large pan over medium heat

- Add sweet potato cubes and cook for about 5 min until slightly tender

- Add red onion and kale, cook for 3 min until kale starts to wilt

- Stir in soy sauce, maple syrup, apple cider vinegar, smoked paprika, salt, and pepper, cook until all vegetables are tender and well-coated with the seasoning

- Garnish with toasted sesame seeds before serving

TIPS: Try adding a pinch of cinnamon for a unique twist - This dish pairs wonderfully with grilled chicken or fish

N.V.: Calories: 188, Fat: 6g, Carbs: 30g, Protein: 4g, Sugar: 9g

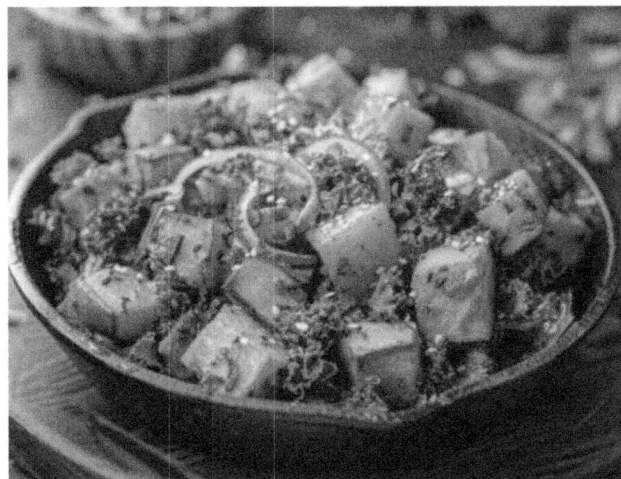

CHAPTER 8: LOW-CARB DAY RECIPES
1. BREAKFAST RECIPES

Low-carb doesn't have to mean low flavor—especially not when it comes to starting your day. Morning meals on low-carb days in The New Carb Cycling System act as your stealthy supporters in the weight management journey, allowing you to enjoy sustained energy without the sugar spike and inevitable crash that higher carb meals can induce.

Picture this: Your day begins with the subtle sizzle of egg and spinach muffins popping out of the oven, their aroma wafting through the air, or perhaps a plate of avocado and bacon omelette lying in wait, its rich textures and flavors promising satisfaction. These breakfast choices aren't just about adhering to a low-carb regimen; they are about crafting experiences that delight both the palate and the body.

Low-carb breakfasts are meticulously designed to integrate seamlessly into your busiest mornings. Whether you are darting out to a meeting or finding that quiet moment before the daily bustle begins, these recipes cater to your lifestyle by being both quick to prepare and profoundly nourishing. Using ingredients that anchor your appetite and stabilize your energy levels, each recipe ensures that you are fully present in whatever task lies ahead.

The real beauty of these low-carb breakfasts lies in their ability to transform simple ingredients into culinary delights. A Greek yogurt parfait, elegantly layered with nuts and seeds, might appear simplistic but is a powerhouse of protein and healthy fats, engineered to keep you full and focused.

So invite optimism into your morning with a breakfast that aligns with your low-carb days but elevates your mealtime to an event that celebrates health and well-being. The journey to weight loss is laden with missteps and challenges, but your first meal of the day should always feel like a victory—an enjoyable, delicious victory that sets a triumphant tone for the hours to come. Through mindful eating and delicious creativity, we can turn each low-carb breakfast into a step toward success.

EGG AND SPINACH MUFFINS

SMOKED SALMON AND SPINACH FRITTATA MUFFINS

P.T.: 15 min | **C.T.:** 20 min

M. of C.: Baking | **SERVES:** 6

INGR: 4 oz. smoked salmon, finely chopped

- 1 C. fresh spinach, roughly chopped

- 6 large eggs

- 1/4 C. heavy cream

- 1/2 C. feta cheese, crumbled

- 2 Tbls fresh dill, chopped

- Salt and pepper to taste

- Non-stick cooking spray

PROC: Preheat oven to 375°F (190°C)

- In a mixing bowl, whisk together eggs, heavy cream, salt, and pepper

- Fold in smoked salmon, spinach, feta cheese, and dill

- Spray a muffin tin with non-stick spray and evenly distribute the mixture into the cups

- Bake for 20 min or until the tops are set and edges are slightly golden

TIPS: Serve immediately or store in an airtight container for up to 3 days - Combine with a side of mixed greens for a perfect low-carb breakfast or lunch

N.V.: Calories: 180, Fat: 13g, Carbs: 2g, Protein: 12g, Sugar: 1g

CHORIZO AND EGG WHITE MUFFINS

P.T.: 10 min | **C.T.:** 18 min

M. of C.: Baking | **SERVES:** 8

INGR: 1/2 lb chorizo, casing removed and crumbled

- 1 C. egg whites

- 1/2 C. red bell pepper, diced

- 1/4 C. onion, finely chopped

- 1/2 tsp ground cumin

- Salt and pepper to taste

- Olive oil spray

PROC: Preheat oven to 375°F (190°C)

- Sauté chorizo, bell pepper, and onion over medium heat until chorizo is browned and vegetables are tender

- Drain and let cool

- In a separate bowl, mix egg whites, cumin, salt, and pepper

- Add cooked chorizo mixture to egg whites and stir to combine

- Spray a muffin pan with olive oil spray and pour the mixture into the cups

- Bake for 18 min or until the muffins are firm to the touch

TIPS: These muffins can be frozen for up to a month for quick breakfast options - Perfect for meal prep - Add a dash of hot sauce for an extra kick

N.V.: Calories: 150, Fat: 8g, Carbs: 3g, Protein: 15g, Sugar: 2g

KALE AND PARMESAN EGG MUFFINS

P.T.: 12 min | **C.T.:** 22 min

M. of C.: Baking | **SERVES:** 6

INGR: 1 C. kale, stems removed and leaves finely chopped

- 6 large eggs

- 1/4 C. milk

- 1/3 C. Parmesan cheese, grated

- 1/4 tsp nutmeg

- Salt and pepper to taste

- Olive oil for greasing

PROC: Preheat oven to 350°F (175°C)

- Blanch kale in boiling water for 2 min, then drain and squeeze out excess water

- Whisk eggs, milk, nutmeg, salt, and pepper in a bowl

- Stir in blanched kale and grated Parmesan

- Grease muffin tin with olive oil and pour the egg mixture evenly into the muffin cups

- Bake for 22 min or until the muffins are set and lightly golden on top

TIPS: Serve with a spoonful of ricotta on top for extra creaminess - Great for a quick snack or paired with a salad for a light meal

N.V.: Calories: 130, Fat: 8g, Carbs: 2g, Protein: 10g, Sugar: 1g

SHIITAKE MUSHROOM AND GRUYERE EGG MUFFINS

P.T.: 10 min | **C.T.:** 25 min

M. of C.: Baking | **SERVES:** 6

INGR: 1/2 C. shiitake mushrooms, thinly sliced

- 6 eggs

- 1/4 C. Gruyere cheese, shredded

- 1/4 C. green onions, sliced

- 1 Tbls olive oil

- Salt and pepper to taste

- Butter for greasing

PROC: Preheat oven to 375°F (190°C)

- Heat olive oil in a skillet over medium heat and sauté shiitake mushrooms until tender

- In a bowl, beat eggs with salt and pepper

- Add cooked mushrooms, Gruyere, and green onions to the egg mixture

- Butter muffin cups and divide the egg mixture among them

- Bake for 25 min or until eggs are set and the tops are slightly browned

TIPS: These muffins are perfect for a portable breakfast or a quick protein boost after a workout - Store in the fridge and just reheat when needed - Pair with a dollop of sour cream for a decadent touch

N.V.: Calories: 140, Fat: 10g, Carbs: 2g, Protein: 11g, Sugar: 1g

AVOCADO AND BACON OMELETTE

CLASSIC AVOCADO AND BACON OMELETTE

P.T.: 10 min. | **C.T.:** 8 min.

M. of C.: Frying | **SERVES:** 1

INGR: 3 eggs, beaten

- 1 ripe avocado, sliced

- 2 slices of nitrate-free bacon, cooked and crumbled

- ¼ C. shredded cheddar cheese

- 1 Tbls olive oil

- Salt and pepper to taste

- 1 Tbls chopped fresh chives

PROC: Heat olive oil in a skillet over medium heat

- Pour in beaten eggs and cook until edges start to lift from the pan

- Add sliced avocado, crumbled bacon, and cheddar cheese on one half of the omelette

- Season with salt and pepper

- Gently fold the omelette over the filling and continue cooking for another 2-3 min. until the cheese melts and the eggs are cooked through

- Serve hot garnished with fresh chives

TIPS: Use a non-stick skillet for easier flipping and less oil - If you like a spicy kick, add a dash of chili flakes before folding the omelette

N.V.: Calories: 485, Fat: 40g, Carbs: 9g, Protein: 27g, Sugar: 2g

ZESTY LIME AND AVOCADO OMELETTE

P.T.: 12 min. | **C.T.:** 7 min.

M. of C.: Frying | **SERVES:** 1

INGR: 3 eggs, beaten

- ½ avocado, diced

- 1 Tbls fresh lime juice

- 2 Tbls finely chopped red onion

- 1 small jalapeño, seeded and finely chopped

- ¼ C. crumbled feta cheese

- Salt and pepper to taste

- 1 Tbls coconut oil

PROC: Heat coconut oil in a skillet over medium-high heat

- Mix avocado, lime juice, red onion, jalapeño, and feta in a bowl

- Pour beaten eggs into the skillet

- As eggs begin to set, spoon the avocado mixture over half of the omelette - Season with salt and pepper

- Fold the omelette over the filling

- Reduce heat to medium-low and cook for further 3 min. until the eggs are fully set and the filling is heated through

TIPS: Serve immediately with a side of fresh salsa for added flavor - Garnish with cilantro for an extra fresh taste

N.V.: Calories: 410, Fat: 32g, Carbs: 12g, Protein: 20g, Sugar: 3g

BACON, AVOCADO, AND GOAT CHEESE OMELETTE

P.T.: 15 min. | **C.T.:** 10 min.

M. of C.: Frying | **SERVES:** 1

INGR: 3 eggs, beaten

- ¼ avocado, sliced

- 3 slices of cooked bacon, chopped

- 2 Tbls goat cheese, crumbled

- 1 Tbls unsalted butter

- Spinach leaves, a handful

- Salt and pepper to taste

- Fresh basil for garnish

PROC: Melt butter in a frying pan over medium heat

- Add beaten eggs and let them set slightly

- Layer the spinach leaves, chopped bacon, sliced avocado, and crumbled goat cheese over half of the omelette

- Season with salt and pepper

- Carefully fold the other half over the filled side

- Cook until the eggs are golden and the filling is warm

- Garnish with fresh basil before serving

TIPS: Adding a few slices of tomato inside can enhance moisture and freshness - Use high-quality goat cheese for creaminess and flavor depth

N.V.: Calories: 495, Fat: 39g, Carbs: 8g, Protein: 29g, Sugar: 2g

GREEK YOGURT WITH NUTS AND SEEDS

VANILLA ALMOND CRUNCH YOGURT

P.T.: 5 min. | **C.T.:** 0 min.

M. of C.: No Cooking | **SERVES:** 2

INGR: 1 C. Greek yogurt, full-fat

- 2 Tbls almond slivers, toasted

- 1 Tbls chia seeds

- 1 tsp vanilla extract

- 2 Tbls pumpkin seeds

- 1 Tbls flaxseed meal

- Sweetener of choice to taste

PROC: Combine Greek yogurt with vanilla extract and sweetener in a bowl

- Toss in almond slivers, pumpkin seeds, chia seeds, and flaxseed meal until evenly distributed

- Serve chilled

TIPS: Add a dash of cinnamon for a spiced variation - Use honey or agave for a natural sweetener option - Experiment with different nuts like walnuts or pecans for varied texture

N.V.: Calories: 280, Fat: 18g, Carbs: 12g, Protein: 20g, Sugar: 4g

BERRY NUT YOGURT FIESTA

P.T.: 10 min. | **C.T.:** 0 min.

M. of C.: No Cooking | **SERVES:** 1

INGR: ¾ C. Greek yogurt, full-fat

- ¼ C. blueberries

- ¼ C. raspberries

- 1 Tbls sunflower seeds

- 1 Tbls hemp seeds

- 1 Tbls raw honey

- 1 Tbls sliced almonds

PROC: Mix Greek yogurt with raw honey thoroughly in a serving bowl

- Add blueberries and raspberries on top of the yogurt

- Sprinkle sliced almonds, sunflower seeds, and hemp seeds over the berries

- Chill before serving if desired

TIPS: Use fresh organic berries for enhanced flavor and nutrition - Replace honey with maple syrup if preferred - Chill overnight to enhance the flavors melding together

N.V.: Calories: 310, Fat: 15g, Carbs: 28g, Protein: 18g, Sugar: 20g

TROPICAL YOGURT DELIGHT

P.T.: 8 min. | **C.T.:** 0 min.

M. of C.: No Cooking | **SERVES:** 2

INGR: 1 C. Greek yogurt, full-fat

- ½ banana, sliced

- 1/4 C. diced mango

- 1 Tbls coconut flakes, unsweetened

- 1 Tbls macadamia nuts, chopped

- 2 tsp lime zest

- 1 Tbls honey

PROC: In a bowl, combine Greek yogurt with honey and lime zest

- Add sliced banana and diced mango to the mix

- Garnish with coconut flakes and chopped macadamia nuts

- Serve immediately or keep chilled

TIPS: Opt to sprinkle a pinch of ground ginger for a zing - Swap mango with pineapple for a different tropical twist - Lime zest can be increased for extra tanginess

N.V.: Calories: 295, Fat: 14g, Carbs: 30g, Protein: 12g, Sugar: 22g

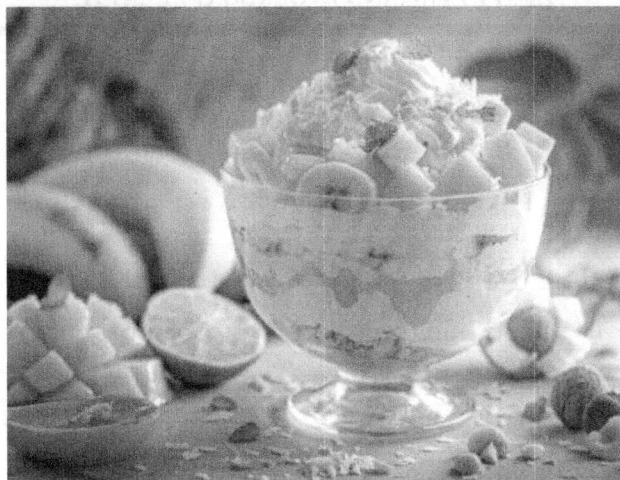

2. LUNCH RECIPES

As we delve into the nuances of low-carb lunch recipes, it's crucial to embrace the diversity and potential these dishes hold for your overall wellness. Transitioning to a midday meal that's low in carbohydrates doesn't mean you're confined to bland or uninspiring choices. Rather, it's an opportunity to explore the rich flavors and textures that ingredients like avocados, leafy greens, and quality proteins bring to the table.

Picture this: a plate with grilled chicken over a vibrant bed of greens, drizzled with a homemade vinaigrette, or perhaps spirals of zucchini noodles delicately tossed with a pesto bursting with fresh basil and pine nuts. These dishes are constructed not only to satisfy your hunger but to fuel your body efficiently, keeping those carb cravings at bay while catering to your bustling schedule.

What's magical about these recipes is their dual ability to align with your weight management goals while fitting effortlessly into a busy lifestyle. They are quick to assemble, yet each bite is packed with nutritional value, ensuring you stay energized without the heft of heavy carbs. This way, your focus remains sharp, and your body nimble, whether you're heading into a critical meeting or picking up the kids from school.

Moreover, these lunches carry the promise of versatility. They can be easily adapted to suit any dietary need or preference, making them perfect for family meals where tastes may vary. Each recipe is a testament to the fact that low-carb eating can indeed be both fulfilling and delicious.

As you explore these recipes, consider them as stepping stones towards a more mindful way of eating, where every meal is an opportunity to nourish not just the body but also the soul. Embracing low-carb lunches is not just about cutting back, but rather enriching your diet with meals that are as delightful as they are wholesome. Now, let's turn the page and discover how satisfying low-carb dining can be.

GRILLED CHICKEN CAESAR SALAD

GRILLED CHICKEN CAESAR SALAD

P.T.: 15 min | **C.T.:** 10 min

M. of C.: Grilling | **SERVES:** 2

INGR: 2 boneless chicken breasts

- 1 tsp garlic powder

- 1 tsp Italian seasoning

- Salt and pepper to taste

- 1 large romaine lettuce, washed and chopped

- 2 Tbls Parmesan cheese, shaved

- 2 Tbls Caesar dressing, low-fat

- 1 lemon, wedged

- 4 anchovy fillets, optional

PROC: Season chicken breasts with garlic powder, Italian seasoning, salt, and pepper

- Preheat grill to medium-high heat (around 375°F or 190°C) and grill chicken until fully cooked and juices run clear, about 5 min per side

- Let chicken rest for 5 min before slicing

- Toss chopped romaine lettuce with Caesar dressing, top with sliced grilled chicken, shaved Parmesan, anchovy fillets if using, and squeeze lemon wedge over salad

TIPS: Grill chicken ahead and refrigerate for a quick salad assembly - Use a vegetable peeler to shave curls of Parmesan directly over the salad - Add croutons if desired, keeping in mind the carb content

N.V.: Calories: 310, Fat: 14g, Carbs: 8g, Protein: 38g, Sugar: 3g

CAESAR-STYLE KALE SALAD WITH GRILLED SHRIMP

P.T.: 20 min | **C.T.:** 8 min

M. of C.: Grilling | **SERVES:** 2

INGR: 12 large shrimp, peeled and deveined

- 1 Tbls olive oil

- 1 tsp smoked paprika

- Salt and black pepper to taste

- 4 cups kale, stems removed and leaves finely chopped

- 2 Tbls Caesar dressing, low-fat

- 1 Tbls Parmesan cheese, grated

- 1 Tbls pine nuts, toasted

- 1 tsp lemon zest

- 1/2 lemon, juiced

PROC: Marinate shrimp in olive oil, smoked paprika, salt, and pepper for 10 min

- Preheat grill to medium-high (375°F or 190°C)

- Grill shrimp until opaque and cooked through, about 3-4 min per side

- Combine chopped kale, Caesar dressing, lemon juice, and zest in a bowl and toss well

- Top kale salad with grilled shrimp, sprinkle with grated Parmesan and toasted pine nuts

TIPS: Toast pine nuts in a dry skillet until golden for added flavor and crunch - Swap kale for baby spinach for a milder taste - Add avocado slices for extra creaminess and healthy fats

N.V.: Calories: 295, Fat: 18g, Carbs: 9g, Protein: 24g, Sugar: 2g

SEARED TUNA CAESAR SALAD

P.T.: 20 min | **C.T.:** 6 min

M. of C.: Searing | **SERVES:** 2

INGR: 2 tuna steaks, about 6 oz each

- 1 Tbls olive oil

- Salt and pepper to taste

- 1 tsp dried herbes de Provence

- 1 romaine lettuce heart, chopped

- 2 Tbls Caesar dressing, low-fat

- 1 Tbls Parmesan cheese, shaved

- 4 cherry tomatoes, halved

- 1/2 red onion, thinly sliced

PROC: Season tuna steaks with salt, pepper, and herbes de Provence

- Heat olive oil in a skillet over high heat and sear tuna steaks about 2-3 min per side for medium-rare

- Slice seared tuna thinly

- Toss chopped romaine with Caesar dressing, arrange on plates, and top with sliced tuna, cherry tomatoes, red onion, and shaved Parmesan

TIPS: Avoid overcooking the tuna to maintain moisture and texture - Sprinkle a little extra herbes de Provence on the salad for enhanced flavor - Pair this dish with a crisp white wine to complement the robust flavors of the tuna

N.V.: Calories: 320, Fat: 14g, Carbs: 7g, Protein: 40g, Sugar: 3g

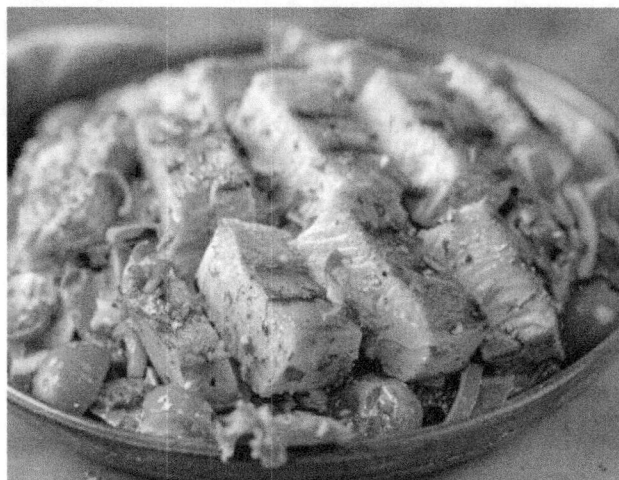

ZUCCHINI NOODLES WITH PESTO

CLASSIC ZUCCHINI NOODLES WITH BASIL PESTO

P.T.: 15 min | **C.T.:** 0 min

M. of C.: No Cooking | **SERVES:** 2

INGR: 2 medium zucchini, spiralized

- 1/2 C. fresh basil leaves

- 1/4 C. pine nuts

- 2 cloves garlic, crushed

- 1/3 C. extra-virgin olive oil

- 1/4 C. Parmesan cheese, grated

- Salt and pepper to taste

PROC: Spiralize zucchini and set aside

- Combine basil, pine nuts, and garlic in a food processor and pulse until coarsely chopped

- Gradually add olive oil while processing until smooth

- Stir in Parmesan, salt, and pepper

- Toss zucchini noodles with pesto until well coated

TIPS: Serve immediately to prevent noodles from becoming soggy - Enhance flavor with a squeeze of fresh lemon juice - Garnish with additional pine nuts and Parmesan if desired

N.V.: Calories: 290, Fat: 26g, Carbs: 8g, Protein: 6g, Sugar: 4g

AVOCADO PESTO ZUCCHINI NOODLES

P.T.: 20 min | **C.T.:** 0 min

M. of C.: No Cooking | **SERVES:** 2

INGR: 2 large zucchini, spiralized

- 1 ripe avocado

- 1/2 C. fresh basil leaves

- 1/4 C. walnuts

- 2 Tbls lemon juice

- 1 clove garlic

- 1/4 C. olive oil

- Salt and pepper to taste

PROC: Spiralize zucchini and place in a bowl

- Blend avocado, basil, walnuts, lemon juice, and garlic in a food processor until smooth

- With the processor running, slowly add olive oil until emulsified

- Season with salt and pepper

- Toss zucchini noodles with avocado pesto until evenly coated

TIPS: Keep the avocado seed in the pesto until serving to prevent browning - Add chili flakes for a spicy kick - Top with cherry tomatoes for added freshness and color

N.V.: Calories: 320, Fat: 27g, Carbs: 12g, Protein: 3g, Sugar: 2g

SUN-DRIED TOMATO AND ALMOND PESTO ZUCCHINI NOODLES

P.T.: 18 min | **C.T.:** 0 min

M. of C.: No Cooking | **SERVES:** 2

INGR: 2 zucchini, spiralized

- 1/3 C. sun-dried tomatoes, oil-packed

- 1/4 C. almonds, toasted

- 1/4 C. Parmesan cheese

- 1/2 cup basil leaves

- 2 Tbls extra-virgin olive oil

- 1 Tbls balsamic vinegar

- Salt to taste

PROC: Spiralize zucchini and set aside

- Blend sun-dried tomatoes, almonds, Parmesan, and basil in a food processor until mixed

- While blending, slowly add olive oil and balsamic vinegar until the mixture forms a coarse paste

- Season with salt

- Toss zucchini noodles with the sun-dried tomato pesto until fully coated

TIPS: Serve topped with additional chopped almonds for crunch - Drizzle with olive oil before serving for extra richness - Pair with grilled chicken or fish for a complete meal

N.V.: Calories: 315, Fat: 25g, Carbs: 15g, Protein: 8g, Sugar: 8g

TUNA SALAD LETTUCE WRAPS

CLASSIC TUNA SALAD LETTUCE WRAPS

P.T.: 15 min | **C.T.:** 0 min

M. of C.: No cooking | **SERVES:** 4

INGR: 2 cans (12 oz each) tuna in water, drained

- 1/2 C. Greek yogurt, plain

- 1/4 C. celery, finely chopped

- 1/4 C. red onion, finely diced

- 2 Tbls fresh dill, chopped

- 1 Tbs capers, rinsed and chopped

- 1 tsp Dijon mustard

- Juice of 1/2 a lemon

- Salt and pepper to taste

- 8 large lettuce leaves, such as Bibb or Romaine

PROC: In a large bowl, combine drained tuna, Greek yogurt, celery, red onion, dill, capers, Dijon mustard, and lemon juice

- Season with salt and pepper to taste

- Mix until all ingredients are evenly distributed

- Spoon the tuna mixture into the center of each lettuce leaf, folding the leaves gently around the filling to form wraps

TIPS: Serve immediately for the freshest taste - For a spicy kick, add a dash of chili flakes or a few drops of hot sauce to the tuna mixture before wrapping - If preparing in advance, store the tuna salad separately and assemble the wraps just before serving

N.V.: Calories: 180, Fat: 2g, Carbs: 3g, Protein: 27g, Sugar: 2g

MEDITERRANEAN TUNA LETTUCE WRAPS

P.T.: 20 min | **C.T.:** 0 min

M. of C.: No cooking | **SERVES:** 4

INGR: 2 cans (12 oz each) tuna in olive oil, drained

- 1/2 C. chopped kalamata olives

- 1/4 C. sun-dried tomatoes, finely chopped

- 1/4 C. feta cheese, crumbled

- 2 Tbls fresh parsley, chopped

- 1 Tbls extra virgin olive oil

- 1 Tbls red wine vinegar

- 1 clove garlic, minced

- Salt and pepper to taste

- 8 large lettuce leaves, such as butter or iceberg

PROC: Combine tuna, kalamata olives, sun-dried tomatoes, feta cheese, parsley, olive oil, red wine vinegar, and minced garlic in a bowl

- Season with salt and pepper to your liking

- Mix thoroughly until all components are well incorporated

- Spoon an even amount of the tuna mixture onto each lettuce leaf

- Wrap the lettuce around the filling to create a neat bundle

TIPS: Add a squeeze of lemon juice for extra zest - These wraps can be paired with a side of quinoa for a more filling meal - Keep the ingredients chilled and assemble just before serving to maintain crispness

N.V.: Calories: 210, Fat: 14g, Carbs: 9g, Protein: 15g, Sugar: 4g

ASIAN ZEST TUNA LETTUCE WRAPS

P.T.: 18 min | **C.T.:** 0 min

M. of C.: No cooking | **SERVES:** 4

INGR: 2 cans (12 oz each) tuna in water, drained

- 1/2 C. carrot, finely shredded

- 1/4 C. cucumber, finely diced

- 1/4 C. red bell pepper, finely diced

- 2 Tbls green onions, sliced

- 2 Tbls cilantro, chopped

- 1 Tbls hoisin sauce

- 1 tsp sesame oil

- 1 tsp freshly grated ginger

- 2 tsp soy sauce (low sodium)

- 8 Iceberg lettuce leaves

PROC: In a mixing bowl, toss together drained tuna, carrot, cucumber, red bell pepper, green onions, and cilantro

- Add hoisin sauce, sesame oil, grated ginger, and soy sauce to the tuna mixture

- Stir gently until all ingredients are evenly mixed

- Place a portion of the tuna mixture into each lettuce leaf and fold or wrap the leaves around the mixture to serve

TIPS: To enhance flavors, let the filling marinate for about 10 min before serving - Sprinkle toasted sesame seeds on top for a crunchy texture - If available, add a few drops of chili oil for a spicy version

N.V.: Calories: 165, Fat: 5g, Carbs: 9g, Protein: 20g, Sugar: 3g

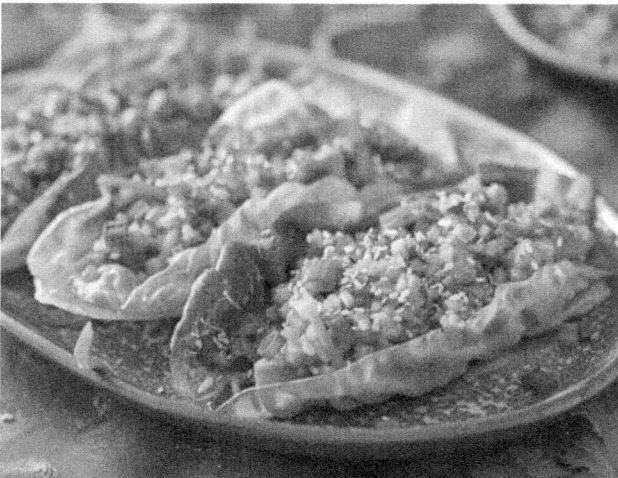

3. Dinner Recipes

Transitioning to a low-carb regimen as the evening shadows grow long might seem like a culinary challenge, yet it's an opportunity to delight in the lighter, yet robust flavors that characterize our low-carb dinner recipes. Evenings are when we seek comfort, a soothing ritual of preparing dishes that don't weigh us down but nourish deeply and prepare us for restful slumber. The recipes in this section have been designed to ensure that your low-carb choices remain diverse and delightful, blending simplicity with nutritional density in ways that might just redefine your notion of dinner.

Consider the end of your day: the need for a meal that caters to unwinding and rejuvenation. Our low-carb dinners such as the herb-crusted chicken breast, beef and broccoli stir-fry, and a surprisingly satisfying cauliflower rice with shrimp, are perfect for those who wish to maintain a light but fulfilling dinner menu. Each recipe is not just crafted to adhere to your dietary needs, but also to fit seamlessly into your lifestyle, capable of being whipped up after a long day's work without sacrificing flavor or quality.

These dishes are woven with ingredients that promote a night of good rest, with proteins to repair and grow muscle while you sleep and fibers to keep your night-time metabolism at just the right pace. The vision behind each dish is to offer a taste experience that satisfies the palate without stretching the carb count, ensuring every dinner is a peaceful nod to your health journey.

Imagine, if you will, plating the herb-crusted chicken breast with a side of aromatic steamed vegetables, or stirring together a colorful, fragrant cauliflower rice with shrimp, each bite a statement of taste yet a whisper in carbs. Such meals promise not just nutritional adequacy but a beautiful end to your day, proving that low-carb can indeed be synonymous with high flavor.

These recipes are your evening companions in the low-carb journey, promising satisfaction at the dinner table without compromising on your dietary goals, ensuring that every night is a step forward in your health quest. Here's to dinners that dovetail perfectly with peaceful evenings and a lifestyle geared towards holistic well-being.

Herb-Crusted Chicken Breast

Rosemary Almond-Crusted Chicken Breast

P.T.: 15 min | **C.T.:** 25 min

M. of C.: Baking | **SERVES:** 4

INGR: 4 boneless, skinless chicken breasts

- 1 C. almond flour

- 2 Tbls fresh rosemary, finely chopped

- 2 cloves garlic, minced

- 1 tsp sea salt

- ½ tsp black pepper

- 2 Tbls Dijon mustard

- 1 Tbls olive oil

PROC: Pat chicken breasts dry with a paper towel

- Season both sides with salt and pepper

- Mix almond flour, rosemary, and minced garlic in a shallow dish

- Brush each chicken breast with Dijon mustard, then press into the almond mixture to coat thoroughly

- Heat olive oil in a skillet over medium heat and sear the chicken on both sides until golden, about 3 min per side

- Transfer to a baking dish and bake in preheated oven at 375°F (190°C) until the chicken reaches an internal temperature of 165°F (74°C), about 15-20 min

TIPS: Let the chicken rest for 5 min before slicing to retain juices - Serve with a side of steamed green beans for a complete meal

N.V.: Calories: 310, Fat: 15g, Carbs: 4g, Protein: 38g, Sugar: 1g

LEMON-THYME CHICKEN WITH HERB CRUST

P.T.: 20 min | **C.T.:** 30 min

M. of C.: Roasting | **SERVES:** 4

INGR: 4 boneless, skinless chicken breasts

- 1 C. crushed pistachios

- 1 Tbls thyme, finely chopped

- Zest of 1 lemon

- 1 tsp sea salt

- ½ tsp cracked black pepper

- 2 Tbls coconut oil

- 2 Tbls lemon juice

PROC: Combine crushed pistachios, thyme, lemon zest, salt, and pepper in a bowl

- Brush each chicken breast with lemon juice then coat uniformly with the pistachio mixture

- Heat coconut oil in an oven-safe skillet over medium-high heat

- Add chicken and sear until each side is golden, approximately 4 min per side

- Transfer skillet to preheated oven at 400°F (204°C) and roast until chicken reaches an internal temperature of 165°F (74°C), about 15-20 min

TIPS: Accompany with roasted asparagus for added flavor and nutrients - Squeeze extra lemon over cooked chicken for a zesty finish

N.V.: Calories: 345, Fat: 19g, Carbs: 6g, Protein: 36g, Sugar: 2g

PARMESAN & SAGE CHICKEN CUTLETS

P.T.: 10 min | **C.T.:** 15 min

M. of C.: Pan-frying | **SERVES:** 4

INGR: 4 chicken cutlets, about 1/4 inch thick

- 1/2 C. Parmesan cheese, grated

- 1/4 C. fresh sage, finely chopped

- 1 clove garlic, minced

- 1 tsp sea salt

- 1/2 tsp black pepper

- 2 Tbls extra-virgin olive oil

PROC: Combine Parmesan, sage, minced garlic, salt, and pepper in a shallow dish

- Press each chicken cutlet into the Parmesan mixture to coat both sides evenly

- Heat olive oil in a large skillet over medium heat

- Fry the chicken cutlets until golden brown and cooked through, about 3-4 min on each side

TIPS: Pair with a light arugula salad tossed in olive oil and lemon dressing for a refreshing contrast - Use freshly grated Parmesan for the best flavor and melting

N.V.: Calories: 275, Fat: 14g, Carbs: 1g, Protein: 32g, Sugar: 0g

BEEF AND BROCCOLI STIR-FRY

SZECHUAN BEEF AND BROCCOLI STIR-FRY

P.T.: 15 min | **C.T.:** 10 min

M. of C.: Stir-Frying | **SERVES:** 4

INGR: 1 lb. flank steak, thinly sliced against the grain

- 2 C. broccoli florets, blanched

- 1 Tbls sesame oil

- 2 garlic cloves, minced

- 1 Tbls fresh ginger, minced

- 3 Tbls low sodium soy sauce

- 1 Tbls oyster sauce

- 1 tsp chili paste

- 1 tsp erythritol

- ½ tsp Szechuan peppercorns, crushed

- 1 green onion, sliced for garnish

- 1 tsp sesame seeds for garnish

PROC: Heat sesame oil in a wok over medium-high heat

- Add garlic and ginger and fry until fragrant, about 1 min

- Increase heat to high, add steak and stir-fry until it starts to brown, around 3-4 min

- Add broccoli, soy sauce, oyster sauce, chili paste, erythritol, and Szechuan peppercorns

- Stir-fry for another 3-4 min until the broccoli is tender and the beef is cooked through

- Garnish with green onion and sesame seeds

TIPS: Serve immediately for the best flavor and texture

- Can be served over cauliflower rice for an even lower carb meal

N.V.: Calories: 280, Fat: 14g, Carbs: 9g, Protein: 29g, Sugar: 2g

BEEF SHIRATAKI NOODLE STIR-FRY

P.T.: 10 min | **C.T.:** 15 min

M. of C.: Stir-Frying | **SERVES:** 2

INGR: 8 oz. shirataki noodles, rinsed and drained

- ½ lb. beef sirloin, thinly sliced

- 1 Tbls avocado oil

- 1 cup snap peas, trimmed

- 1 bell pepper, julienne

- ½ onion, thinly sliced

- 2 Tbls tamari sauce

- 1 Tbls fish sauce

- 1 Tbls lime juice

- 1 tsp xylitol

- 1 Tbls Thai basil, chopped

- 1 Tbls chili flakes

PROC: Heat oil in a large skillet over medium-high heat

- Add onion and bell pepper and sauté until softened, about 3 min

- Add beef and cook until browned, about 5 min

- Add snap peas, shirataki noodles, tamari, fish sauce, lime juice, and xylitol

- Stir-fry until everything is heated through and coated in sauce, about 5 min

- Remove from heat and stir in Thai basil and chili flakes

TIPS: Perfectly paired with a side of stir-fried bok choy

- Use a high smoke point oil like avocado oil for optimal stir-frying results

N.V.: Calories: 220, Fat: 8g, Carbs: 10g, Protein: 25g, Sugar: 4g

SPICY LEMON GRASS BEEF

P.T.: 20 min | **C.T.:** 10 min

M. of C.: Stir-Frying | **SERVES:** 4

INGR: 1 lb. lean ground beef

- 2 stalks lemongrass, finely minced

- 4 Kaffir lime leaves, finely chopped

- 1 red chili, deseeded and finely sliced

- 1 Tbls fish sauce

- 2 Tbls coconut aminos

- 1 Tbls coconut oil

- 1 tsp stevia

- Juice of 1 lime

- ¼ cup cilantro, chopped for garnish

PROC: Heat coconut oil in a skillet over medium heat

- Add lemongrass, lime leaves, and red chili and sauté until aromatic, about 2 min

- Add ground beef and brown, breaking it up as it cooks, about 8 min

- Stir in fish sauce, coconut aminos, and stevia

- Cook for an additional 2 min

- Remove from heat and squeeze over lime juice

- Garnish with chopped cilantro

TIPS: Serve with leafy greens for a complete meal - Adjust the amount of red chili for desired heat level

N.V.: Calories: 180, Fat: 10g, Carbs: 3g, Protein: 20g, Sugar: 1g

CAULIFLOWER RICE WITH SHRIMP

CAULIFLOWER RICE WITH CITRUS SHRIMP

P.T.: 15 min | **C.T.:** 10 min

M. of C.: Stovetop | **SERVES:** 4

INGR: 1 medium cauliflower head, grated into rice-sized pieces

- 1 lb. shrimp, peeled and deveined

- 2 Tbls extra virgin olive oil

- 1 garlic clove, minced

- Zest and juice of 1 orange

- Zest and juice of 1 lime

- 1/2 tsp red pepper flakes

- 1/4 C. fresh cilantro, chopped

- Salt and black pepper to taste

PROC: Heat olive oil over medium heat in a large skillet

- Add garlic and sauté until fragrant, about 1 min

- Increase heat to medium-high, add shrimp and cook until they turn pink and opaque, about 3-4 min, then remove from pan

- In the same skillet, add cauliflower rice, orange and lime zest, and juice, sautéing until the cauliflower is tender, around 5-6 min

- Return shrimp to skillet, toss with red pepper flakes, cilantro, salt, and black pepper, heat through

TIPS: Use freshly squeezed citrus juice for better flavor - Garnish with additional cilantro for a fresh presentation - Serve warm as a light and refreshing low-carb meal

N.V.: Calories: 250, Fat: 8g, Carbs: 15g, Protein: 25g, Sugar: 6g

GARLIC BUTTER SHRIMP WITH HERBED CAULIFLOWER RICE

P.T.: 20 min | **C.T.:** 15 min

M. of C.: Stovetop | **SERVES:** 2

INGR: 1 small cauliflower, riced

- 1 lb. shrimp, cleaned and deveined

- 4 Tbls unsalted butter

- 1 Tbls garlic, finely chopped

- 1 tsp Italian seasoning

- 1/2 tsp chili flakes

- Salt and pepper to taste

- 2 Tbls parsley, finely chopped

- 1 Tbls lemon juice

PROC: Melt butter over medium heat in a skillet

- Add garlic and sauté until golden, about 1 min

- Add shrimp, sprinkle with Italian seasoning, chili flakes, salt, and pepper, and cook until shrimp are pink, about 3-5 min

- Remove shrimp and set aside

- In the same skillet, add the riced cauliflower, cook until soft, about 7-8 min

- Mix in parsley and lemon juice, return shrimp to skillet, toss well to combine and reheat for 2 min

TIPS: Pair with a side of steamed asparagus for a complete meal - If preferred, sprinkle with grated Parmesan before serving for added flavor

N.V.: Calories: 295, Fat: 18g, Carbs: 10g, Protein: 24g, Sugar: 3g

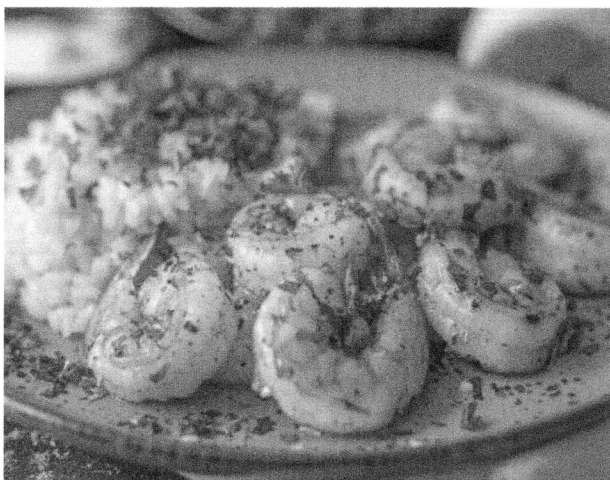

SPICY SHRIMP OVER LIME INFUSED CAULIFLOWER RICE

P.T.: 10 min | **C.T.:** 12 min

M. of C.: Stovetop | **SERVES:** 3

INGR: 1 large cauliflower, pulsed into rice

- 1 lb. shrimp, peeled and deveined

- 1 Tbls coconut oil

- 1/2 tsp cayenne pepper

- 1/2 tsp paprika

- 1 lime, zest and juice

- Salt to taste

- 1/4 C. green onions, sliced

- 1 Tbls fresh mint, chopped

PROC: Heat coconut oil in a skillet over medium-high heat

- Season shrimp with cayenne pepper, paprika, and salt, add to the skillet and cook until they are opaque, about 4-5 min

- Remove shrimp and set aside

- In the same skillet, add cauliflower rice and lime zest, cook until tender, about 5-7 min

- Stir in lime juice, green onions, and mint

- Add shrimp back into the skillet, stir until well combined and heated through

TIPS: Serve immediately for best flavor - The lime zest adds a fresh zing that complements the spicy shrimp beautifully

N.V.: Calories: 215, Fat: 6g, Carbs: 13g, Protein: 26g, Sugar: 4g

CHAPTER 9: MEDIUM-CARB DAY RECIPES
1. BREAKFAST RECIPES

When it comes to the nuanced art of carb cycling, medium-carb days provide a delightful balance—a symphony of flavors and nutrients designed to keep your metabolism finely tuned while catering to your palate's desires. The breakfast recipes in this section embody that delicate equilibrium, striking a perfect balance between fueling your body and indulging your taste buds without going overboard.

Imagine starting your day with a smoothie blended to creamy perfection, with banana and almond butter providing just the right amount of carbs along with a robust dose of protein. Or consider the simple elegance of whole grain toast, topped with creamy avocado and a perfectly poached egg— textures and flavors that marry convenience with health benefits.

These recipes are crafted for those days when your body needs more than the bare minimum but less than the feasts of high-carb days. They understand and cater to your physiological needs, utilizing medium-level carbohydrates to replenish your energy stores adequately after perhaps a more vigorous gym session or a particularly taxing day ahead.

These meals do more than just satiate and nourish; they bring a sense of fulfillment that only food made with care can offer. A berry parfait with Greek yogurt might sound whimsical, but here it serves a serious purpose. It's more than just a delightful dish; it's planned to provide the energy spikes your body needs while still aligning with your goals of weight management and health improvement.

Let each breakfast be an opportunity to moderate, to balance. It's about finding that sweet middle ground in your diet where you can feel satisfied by your meal without feeling weighed down. This section isn't just about recipes—it's a roadmap to smart, deliberate choices that exemplify how a strategic approach to carbohydrate intake can transform not just your body but your relationship with food. Dive into these breakfasts with the confidence that they are steps on a path tailored just for your journey toward health and vitality.

BANANA AND ALMOND BUTTER SMOOTHIE

BANANA AND ALMOND BUTTER SMOOTHIE

P.T.: 5 min. | **C.T.:** 0 min.

M. of C.: Blending | **SERVES:** 2

INGR: 2 ripe bananas, peeled and sliced

- 2 Tbls almond butter

- 1 C. unsweetened almond milk

- ½ C. Greek yogurt

- 1 Tbls honey

- 1 tsp ground cinnamon

- ½ tsp vanilla extract

- 4 ice cubes

PROC: Place bananas, almond butter, almond milk, Greek yogurt, honey, cinnamon, vanilla extract, and ice cubes in a blender

- Blend on high until smooth and creamy

TIPS: Serve immediately for the best flavor and consistency - Adjust sweetness by adding more honey if desired - Add a scoop of vanilla protein powder for an extra protein boost

N.V.: Calories: 295, Fat: 11g, Carbs: 44g, Protein: 8g, Sugar: 30g

SPICY BANANA ALMOND SHAKE

P.T.: 7 min. | **C.T.:** 0 min.

M. of C.: Blending | **SERVES:** 1

INGR: 1 large banana, frozen and chopped

- 1 Tbls almond butter

- 1 C. oat milk

- 1 tsp chia seeds

- 1/4 tsp cayenne pepper

- Pinch of nutmeg

- 1 tsp maple syrup

PROC: Combine all ingredients in a high-powered blender

- Blend until the mixture is smooth and the chia seeds are fully incorporated, resulting in a thick consistency

TIPS: This shake can be thinned with additional oat milk if needed - The cayenne pepper adds a warming kick, which can be adjusted to taste - Ideal as a rejuvenating post-workout drink

N.V.: Calories: 280, Fat: 9g, Carbs: 45g, Protein: 5g, Sugar: 22g

NUTTY BANANA BLENDER PANCAKES

P.T.: 10 min. | **C.T.:** 5 min.

M. of C.: Griddling | **SERVES:** 2

INGR: 2 ripe bananas

- 1 C. oat flour

- 1 Tbls almond butter

- 2 eggs

- 1/2 tsp baking powder

- Pinch of salt

- 1/4 C. almond milk

- Cooking spray

PROC: In a blender, mix bananas, almond butter, eggs, oat flour, baking powder, salt, and almond milk until smooth

- Heat a non-stick skillet over medium heat and coat with cooking spray

- Pour batter to form pancakes, cooking until bubbles form on top, then flip to cook other side

TIPS: Serve hot with a dollop of Greek yogurt and a drizzle of honey - Experiment by adding blueberries or chocolate chips to the batter for a twist - These pancakes store well in the refrigerator for quick breakfast options

N.V.: Calories: 320, Fat: 12g, Carbs: 44g, Protein: 10g, Sugar: 15g

WHOLE GRAIN TOAST WITH AVOCADO AND EGGS

SAVORY AVOCADO TOAST WITH POACHED EGG AND ARUGULA

P.T.: 10 min | **C.T.:** 6 min

M. of C.: Stovetop | **SERVES:** 1

INGR: 1 slice whole grain sourdough

- 1 ripe avocado

- 1 large organic egg

- 1 Tbls white vinegar

- ¼ C. fresh arugula

- 1 tsp lemon juice

- Salt and black pepper to taste

- 1 pinch chili flakes

- 1 Tbls extra virgin olive oil

PROC: Fill a pot with water, add vinegar, and bring to a simmer

- Crack egg into a cup and gently pour into simmering water

- Poach for about 3-4 min until whites are set but yolk remains runny

- Mash avocado with lemon juice, salt, and pepper

- Toast whole grain sourdough till golden

- Spread mashed avocado on toast, top with poached egg, arugula, drizzle with olive oil, and sprinkle with chili flakes

TIPS: For a creamier texture, blend avocado with a splash of Greek yogurt

- To avoid breaking the yolk, use a fresh egg as they hold their shape better in simmering water - Squeeze a dash of lime over the top for an extra zest

N.V.: Calories: 290, Fat: 19g, Carbs: 24g, Protein: 12g, Sugar: 2g

EGG-OCADO TOAST WITH CHERRY TOMATOES AND FETA

P.T.: 15 min | **C.T.:** 10 min

M. of C.: Oven | **SERVES:** 1

INGR: 1 slice multigrain bread

- 1 ripe avocado

- 1 large egg

- 5 cherry tomatoes, halved

- 2 Tbls crumbled feta cheese

- Salt and pepper to taste

- 1 Tbls fresh chopped basil

- 1 tsp olive oil

PROC: Preheat oven to 360°F (182°C)

- Slice avocado and lay it on bread, creating a well in the center

- Crack an egg into the well

- Top with tomatoes and feta

- Season with salt and pepper

- Bake for about 10 min until egg whites are set

- Remove, sprinkle with basil, and drizzle with olive oil

TIPS: Serve immediately for best texture of egg - Adding a sprinkle of red pepper flakes gives a spicy kick - A drizzle of balsamic reduction can intensify the flavors

N.V.: Calories: 320, Fat: 20g, Carbs: 27g, Protein: 13g, Sugar: 5g

CAPRESE AVOCADO TOAST WITH SOFT BOILED EGG

P.T.: 12 min | **C.T.:** 7 min

M. of C.: Stovetop | **SERVES:** 2

INGR: 2 slices of whole grain ciabatta

- 1 large avocado

- 2 large eggs

- 4 slices fresh mozzarella

- 6 slices ripe Roma tomato

- Balsamic glaze

- Fresh basil leaves

- Salt and black pepper to taste

- 1 Tbls olive oil

PROC: Bring water to a boil, gently add eggs and boil for exactly 7 min for a soft yolk

- Peel eggs under cold water

- Toast ciabatta slices until crispy

- Mash avocado with salt and pepper and spread on toasted bread

- Layer with mozzarella slices and tomato

- Halve soft-boiled eggs and place over the top

- Garnish with basil leaves, a drizzle of olive oil, and balsamic glaze

TIPS: Soft boiled eggs can also be made ahead of time and stored in cold water to maintain freshness - Rubbing garlic on the toasted ciabatta before adding avocado can enhance flavor - A sprinkle of coarse sea salt will elevate the layers of taste

N.V.: Calories: 410, Fat: 27g, Carbs: 29g, Protein: 18g, Sugar: 3g

BERRY PARFAIT WITH GREEK YOGURT

MATCHA BERRY PARFAIT WITH GREEK YOGURT

P.T.: 15 min | **C.T.:** 0 min

M. of C.: No Cooking | **SERVES:** 2

INGR: 1 C. Greek yogurt, plain

- 1 Tbls matcha powder

- ½ C. mixed berries (blueberries, raspberries)

- ¼ C. granola

- 1 Tbls honey

- 2 tsp chia seeds

PROC: Combine Greek yogurt with matcha powder in a bowl and mix until uniformly green

- In serving glasses, layer a spoonful of matcha yogurt, then a layer of mixed berries, sprinkle some granola and a little chia seeds, repeat layering until glasses are filled

- Drizzle honey over the top layer

TIPS: Serve immediately or chill for an hour for flavors to meld - Opt for organic honey for enhanced flavor - Try adding a pinch of lemon zest to the yogurt for a citrusy twist

N.V.: Calories: 220, Fat: 5g, Carbs: 35g, Protein: 12g, Sugar: 20g

FIG AND PISTACHIO GREEK YOGURT PARFAIT

P.T.: 10 min | **C.T.:** 0 min

M. of C.: No Cooking | **SERVES:** 2

INGR: 1 C. Greek yogurt, plain

- 4 fresh figs, quartered

- ¼ C. pistachios, crushed

- 2 Tbls honey

- 1 tsp vanilla extract

PROC: In a mixing bowl, combine Greek yogurt with vanilla extract

- In serving glasses, alternate layers of yogurt, fresh figs, and crushed pistachios

- Repeat layering until glasses are full

- Drizzle honey uniformly over the top

TIPS: Consider using Greek yogurt with a high protein content for added nutritional benefits - Substitute figs with dates for a different flavor profile - Garnish with a few whole pistachios for a pleasing presentation

N.V.: Calories: 295, Fat: 9g, Carbs: 40g, Protein: 15g, Sugar: 28g

POMEGRANATE AND WALNUT PARFAIT WITH GREEK YOGURT

P.T.: 12 min | **C.T.:** 0 min

M. of C.: No Cooking | **SERVES:** 2

INGR: 1 C. Greek yogurt, plain

- ½ C. pomegranate seeds

- ¼ C. walnuts, toasted and chopped

- 2 Tbls maple syrup

- ½ tsp cinnamon powder

PROC: Toast walnuts lightly in a dry pan, then cool and chop

- Mix Greek yogurt with cinnamon powder

- In serving cups, layer yogurt, pomegranate seeds, and walnuts, repeat the layers until full

- Drizzle with maple syrup before serving

TIPS: Refrigerating for at least 30 min enhances the flavors - Maple syrup can be replaced with agave for a lower glycemic index option - To add texture, sprinkle a few hemp seeds on the top layer just before serving

N.V.: Calories: 270, Fat: 8g, Carbs: 32g, Protein: 14g, Sugar: 22g

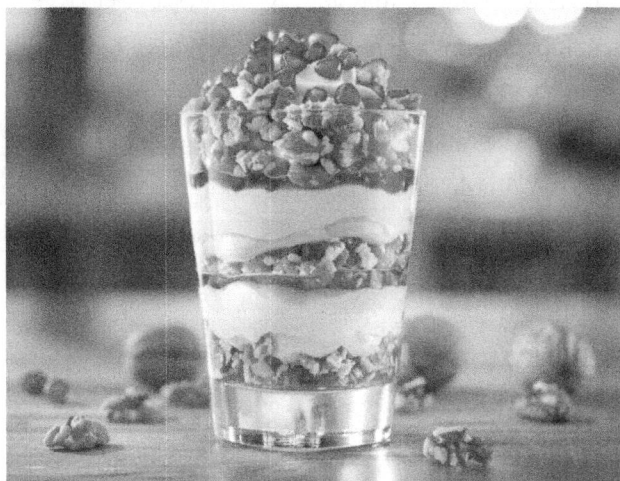

2. Lunch Recipes

Navigating through medium-carb lunch recipes offers a delightful balance that fits perfectly into your carb cycling framework, a golden mean that combines the lightness of lower carb options with the satisfying, energy-sustaining boost found in higher carb meals. It's about harmony – filling yet not overly indulgent, perfectly tuned to support an active lifestyle while facilitating weight management.

Imagine cozying up to a meal that hits that sweet spot: a turkey and quinoa stuffed pepper that's both satiating and nutritiously balanced, or a grilled veggie and hummus wrap that envelops all the richness of flavor and texture you crave without the post-lunch energy dip. These dishes do more than just fill your stomach; they nourish your body and prepare your mind for the challenges of your dynamic afternoon schedule.

It's the flexibility of these medium-carb meals that stands out. They are adaptable for a solo lunch or can be effortlessly scaled up to cater to family or friends on shared meal occasions. This adaptability makes them a resourceful player in your nutritional arsenal, ensuring you can maintain your dietary strategy without feeling restricted by overly strict carb limits.

By providing a balanced spectrum of nutrients from smart carb sources mixed with quality proteins and vibrant veggies, each medium-carb recipe ensures your energy levels remain steady. You can expect to glide through your day with a rejuvenated focus, capable of tackling professional tasks or enjoying personal pursuits with equal zest.

Delve into these recipes with the anticipation of discovery, where each ingredient is selected to enhance your midday meal, ensuring enjoyment and effectiveness in every forkful. This is not just about sticking to a regimen; it's about savoring your way to well-being and productivity. These meals are designed to delight your palate, nourish your body, and align beautifully with your carb cycling journey. Now, let's explore the delicious possibilities that medium-carb can offer!

Turkey and Quinoa Stuffed Peppers

Southwest Turkey and Quinoa Stuffed Peppers

P.T.: 20 min. | **C.T.:** 35 min.

M. of C.: Baking | **SERVES:** 4

INGR: 4 large bell peppers, halved and seeded

- 1 lb. ground turkey

- 1 C. cooked quinoa

- 1 C. black beans, drained and rinsed

- 1 C. corn kernels

- 1 medium onion, diced

- 2 cloves garlic, minced

- 1 tsp. cumin

- 1 tsp. chili powder

- 1/2 tsp. smoked paprika

- 1/4 C. fresh cilantro, chopped

- 1 C. shredded Monterey Jack cheese

- Salt and pepper to taste

PROC: Preheat oven to 375°F (190°C)

- In a skillet, cook ground turkey, onion, and garlic over medium heat until turkey is browned

- Stir in cumin, chili powder, paprika, quinoa, black beans, and corn, cook for an additional 5 min.

- Remove from heat, add cilantro, salt, and pepper

- Stuff the pepper halves with the turkey mix

- Top each with shredded cheese

- Arrange in baking dish

- Cover with foil and bake for 25 min., then uncover and bake for additional 10 min. until peppers are tender and cheese is bubbly

TIPS: Serve with a dollop of sour cream and a sprinkle of chopped scallions for extra flavor - Can be prepared ahead and stored in the refrigerator overnight, enhances flavors

N.V.: Calories: 450, Fat: 22g, Carbs: 35g, Protein: 28g, Sugar: 7g

TURKEY AND QUINOA STUFFED PEPPERS WITH FETA AND SPINACH

P.T.: 20 min. | **C.T.:** 35 min.

M. of C.: Oven Baking | **SERVES:** 4

INGR: 4 large bell peppers, tops removed and seeds discarded

- 1 lb. ground turkey
- 1 C. cooked quinoa
- 1 C. fresh spinach, chopped
- ½ C. crumbled feta cheese
- 1 small onion, finely chopped
- 2 cloves garlic, minced
- 1 tsp dried oregano
- 1 tsp smoked paprika
- Salt and pepper to taste
- 1 Tbls olive oil
- 1 C. tomato sauce
- ½ C. chicken broth

PROC: Preheat oven to 375°F (190°C)

- Heat olive oil in a skillet over medium heat
- Add onion and garlic, sauté until softened
- Stir in ground turkey, cooking until browned
- Mix in quinoa, spinach, feta, oregano, paprika, salt, and pepper
- Stuff each bell pepper with the turkey mixture and place in a baking dish
- Pour tomato sauce and chicken broth around the peppers
- Cover with foil and bake for 30 minutes
- Remove foil and bake an additional 5 minutes or until peppers are tender

TIPS: For a spicier kick, add a pinch of red pepper flakes to the turkey mixture - Serve with a side of steamed vegetables for a complete meal

N.V.: Calories: 310, Fat: 14g, Carbs: 22g, Protein: 27g, Sugar: 6g

TURKEY AND QUINOA STUFFED PEPPERS WITH SUNDRIED TOMATOES AND GOAT CHEESE

P.T.: 25 min. | **C.T.:** 40 min.

M. of C.: Oven Baking | **SERVES:** 4

INGR: 4 large bell peppers, tops removed and seeds discarded

- 1 lb. ground turkey
- 1 C. cooked quinoa
- ½ C. sundried tomatoes, chopped
- 4 oz. goat cheese, crumbled
- 1 small zucchini, grated
- 1 small onion, finely chopped
- 2 cloves garlic, minced
- 1 tsp dried basil
- 1 tsp cumin
- Salt and pepper to taste
- 1 Tbls olive oil
- 1 C. marinara sauce
- ½ C. vegetable broth

PROC: Preheat oven to 375°F (190°C)

- Heat olive oil in a skillet over medium heat
- Add onion and garlic, sauté until softened
- Stir in ground turkey, cooking until browned
- Mix in quinoa, sundried tomatoes, zucchini, goat cheese, basil, cumin, salt, and pepper
- Stuff each bell pepper with the turkey mixture and place in a baking dish
- Pour marinara sauce and vegetable broth around the peppers
- Cover with foil and bake for 35 minutes
- Remove foil and bake an additional 5 minutes or until peppers are tender

TIPS: Try topping with fresh basil leaves before serving for added flavor - Use a mix of red and yellow peppers for a more colorful presentation

N.V.: Calories: 325, Fat: 16g, Carbs: 23g, Protein: 26g, Sugar: 7g

GRILLED VEGGIE AND HUMMUS WRAP

MEDITERRANEAN GRILLED VEGGIE AND HUMMUS WRAP

P.T.: 15 min | **C.T.:** 10 min

M. of C.: Grilling | **SERVES:** 2

INGR: 2 whole wheat tortillas

- 1 zucchini, sliced into ribbons

- 1 bell pepper, julienned

- 1 small red onion, thinly sliced

- 1 Tbls olive oil

- 1 tsp dried oregano

- 1/2 C. hummus

- 1/4 C. feta cheese, crumbled

- 1 handful of fresh arugula

- Salt and pepper to taste

PROC: Preheat grill to medium-high heat (around 375°F (190°C))

- Toss zucchini, bell pepper, and onion with olive oil, oregano, salt, and pepper

- Grill vegetables until tender and slightly charred, about 5-6 min per side

- Warm tortillas on the grill for about 1 min on each side

- Spread hummus on each tortilla, add grilled vegetables, sprinkle feta cheese, and top with arugula

- Roll up tightly, slice in half, and serve

TIPS: Use a grill basket for smaller veggies to prevent them from falling through the grates - Include a drizzle of lemon juice or balsamic reduction for added zest - Pair with a side of Kalamata olives for a true Mediterranean flair

N.V.: Calories: 320, Fat: 15g, Carbs: 40g, Protein: 8g, Sugar: 5g

SPICY THAI PEANUT VEGGIE WRAP

P.T.: 20 min | **C.T.:** 5 min

M. of C.: Pan Searing | **SERVES:** 2

INGR: 2 spinach tortillas

- 1/2 C. shredded carrots

- 1/2 C. thinly sliced red cabbage

- 1/2 C. sliced bell peppers

- 1 green onion, thinly sliced

- 1 Tbls coconut oil

- 1 tsp chili flakes

- 2 Tbls peanut butter

- 1 Tbls hoisin sauce

- 1 tsp soy sauce

- 1 tsp lime juice

- Fresh cilantro for garnish

- Crushed peanuts for topping

- Salt to taste

PROC: Heat coconut oil in a pan over medium heat

- Add carrots, red cabbage, bell peppers, and chili flakes, sauté for 3-4 min until veggies are slightly softened

- In a small bowl, mix peanut butter, hoisin sauce, soy sauce, and lime juice until smooth

- Spread the peanut sauce mixture over each tortilla

- Distribute the cooked veggies on top and sprinkle green onion, cilantro, and crushed peanuts

- Roll tightly, slice in half, and serve

TIPS: Enhance flavor with a sprinkle of sesame seeds - If you prefer a less spicy wrap, reduce the amount of chili flakes or remove them altogether - Perfect for packing as a nutritious lunch

N.V.: Calories: 270, Fat: 14g, Carbs: 32g, Protein: 7g, Sugar: 8g

CALIFORNIA AVOCADO AND SPROUTS WRAP

P.T.: 10 min | **C.T.:** 0 min

M. of C.: No Cooking | **SERVES:** 2

INGR: 2 tomato basil tortillas

- 1 ripe avocado, mashed

- 1/2 C. alfalfa sprouts

- 1/2 cucumber, thinly sliced

- 1/2 C. cherry tomatoes, halved

- 1/4 C. red onion, thinly sliced

- 2 Tbls ranch dressing

- 1 tsp hot sauce

- Salt and pepper to taste

- 1/4 C. shredded Monterey Jack cheese

PROC: Spread mashed avocado evenly over tortillas

- Top with alfalfa sprouts, cucumber slices, cherry tomatoes, and red onion

- In a small dish, combine ranch dressing and hot sauce, drizzle over the veggies

- Sprinkle Monterey Jack cheese on top

- Season with salt and pepper

- Roll up the tortillas tightly, slice in half, and serve

TIPS: Opt for a vegan substitute like cashew-based cheese to make this wrap dairy-free - Add slices of grilled chicken or tofu for extra protein - Wrap can be made ahead and refrigerated until ready to serve

N.V.: Calories: 280, Fat: 18g, Carbs: 26g, Protein: 7g, Sugar: 4g

CHICKEN AND BARLEY SOUP

CHICKEN AND PEARL BARLEY SOUP WITH ROOT VEGETABLES

P.T.: 20 min. | **C.T.:** 1 hr.

M. of C.: Stovetop | **SERVES:** 4

INGR: 2 Tbls olive oil

- 1 lb. skinless chicken thighs, cubed

- 1 C. pearl barley

- 6 C. chicken stock

- 1 C. carrots, diced

- 1 C. parsnips, diced

- 1 C. leeks, thinly sliced

- 2 cloves garlic, minced

- 1 tsp dried thyme

- Salt and pepper to taste

PROC: Heat olive oil in a large pot over medium heat

- Add chicken and cook until browned, about 5 min.

- Add garlic and leeks, sauté until leeks are softened, 3 min.

- Stir in carrots, parsnips, barley, thyme, salt, pepper, and chicken stock

- Bring to a boil, then reduce heat to low and simmer covered until barley is tender, about 50 min.

TIPS: Add a splash of white wine during cooking for enhanced flavor - Serve with a sprinkle of fresh parsley for freshness and color

N.V.: Calories: 345, Fat: 9g, Carbs: 45g, Protein: 24g, Sugar: 5g

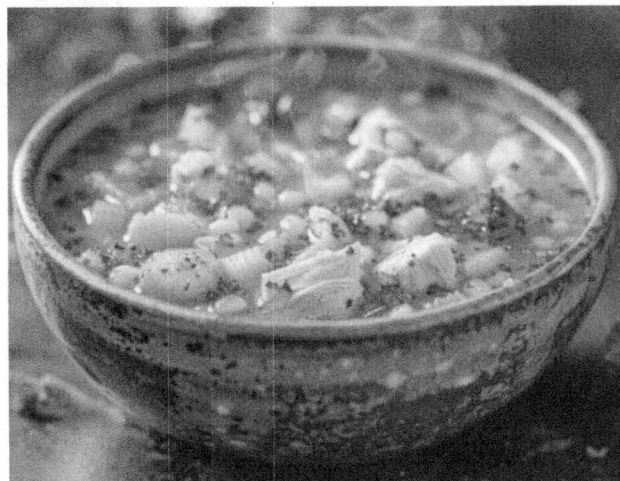

CREAMY CHICKEN AND BARLEY SOUP WITH MUSHROOMS

P.T.: 15 min. | **C.T.:** 40 min.

M. of C.: Stovetop | **SERVES:** 4

INGR: 1 Tbls butter

- 1 lb. chicken breast, diced

- 1 C. barley

- 5 C. mushroom broth

- 1 C. sliced mushrooms

- 1 onion, chopped

- 1 celery stalk, diced

- 2 Tbls heavy cream

- 1 tsp dried sage

- Salt and pepper to taste

PROC: Melt butter in a soup pot over medium heat

- Add chicken, onion, and celery, cook until chicken is browned, about 10 min.

- Mix in mushrooms and cook until tender, 5 min.

- Add barley, sage, salt, pepper, and mushroom broth

- Bring to boil, then reduce heat and simmer until barley is soft, about 25 min.

- Stir in heavy cream just before serving

TIPS: Garnish with chopped chives for an aromatic touch - Use low-fat cream to reduce calories without compromising texture

N.V.: Calories: 360, Fat: 12g, Carbs: 40g, Protein: 25g, Sugar: 3g

SPICY CHICKEN AND BARLEY SOUP WITH KALE

P.T.: 25 min. | **C.T.:** 55 min.

M. of C.: Stovetop | **SERVES:** 6

INGR: 1 Tbls coconut oil

- 1 lb. chicken drumsticks

- 1 C. hulled barley

- 6 C. vegetable broth

- 2 C. kale, chopped

- 1 red bell pepper, diced

- 1 yellow onion, diced

- 2 Tbls tomato paste

- 1 tsp smoked paprika

- 2 tsp chili powder

- 1 tsp cumin

- Salt to taste

PROC: Heat coconut oil in a large saucepan over medium-high heat

- Add onion and bell pepper, sauté until soft, about 8 min.

- Add drumsticks and sear on all sides, about 10 min.

- Stir in tomato paste, paprika, chili powder, cumin, and salt, cook for 2 min.

- Pour in vegetable broth and add barley

- Bring to a simmer, reduce heat to low, cover, and cook until barley is tender, about 35 min.

- Add chopped kale in the last 5 min. of cooking

TIPS: Sprinkle with lime zest for a citrusy lift - Serve with avocado slices for added creaminess and healthy fats

N.V.: Calories: 295, Fat: 8g, Carbs: 38g, Protein: 20g, Sugar: 4g

3. Dinner Recipes

As dusk settles and the hearty laugh of a day well spent fills the air, the dinner table becomes a center stage for balance during our medium-carb days. This chapter is dedicated to those who seek a harmonious blend of flexibility and structure in their nutritional regime. The medium-carb dinner recipes are designed not only to satiate but to stabilize, offering a mid-ground that supports your energy levels without tipping the scales too far in any one direction.

Here, the meals are rich tapestries woven with strands of wholesome grains, lean proteins, and vibrant vegetables. Dishes like baked cod with roasted vegetables, turkey chili, and spaghetti squash with marinara and meatballs stand as pillars of what it means to have a meal that's as nourishing as it is satisfying. These dinners are designed to maintain your momentum, keeping you neither too light nor too weighed down as you head into the evening hours.

Imagine the rich yet balanced aromas filling your kitchen as a spaghetti squash roasts to perfection, later to be paired with a hearty, homemade marinara sauce. Such dishes embrace the spirit of moderation that characterizes medium-carb living, showing how a middle path can also be the most enriching—one that fosters a relationship with food that is freeing rather than constrictive.

These recipes ensure you close your day feeling fulfilled and content, making it easier to maintain your carb cycling without feeling deprived. They are a testament to the fact that balance doesn't have to mean bland; rather, it's a dynamic state where nutrition and pleasure meet effortlessly at the end of your day.

Engage with each recipe as a companion to a lifestyle that cherishes health and happiness in equal measure. Here's to dinners that not only feed the body but also nourish the spirit, providing a balanced plate that satisfies both the taste buds and nutritional needs. As you explore this chapter, let each recipe remind you that in the art of eating well, the middle way is often rich with flavors and possibilities.

Baked Cod with Roasted Vegetables

Baked Cod with Roasted Rainbow Carrots and Parsnips

P.T.: 15 min | **C.T.:** 25 min

M. of C.: Baking | **SERVES:** 4

INGR: 4 6-oz portions of cod fillet

- 2 C. rainbow carrots, peeled and sliced

- 2 C. parsnips, peeled and sliced

- 3 Tbls extra virgin olive oil

- 1 tsp smoked paprika

- 1 tsp garlic powder

- 1 Tbls fresh thyme, chopped

- Sea salt and black pepper to taste

PROC: Preheat oven to 425°F (220°C)

- In a bowl, mix carrots and parsnips with 2 Tbls olive oil, smoked paprika, garlic powder, salt, and pepper

- Spread on a baking tray and roast for 10 min

- Place cod fillets on the tray, drizzle with remaining 1 Tbls olive oil and sprinkle with thyme

- Bake for 15 min or until cod is flaky and vegetables are tender

TIPS: Rotate vegetables halfway through for even cooking - Pair with a side of quinoa for a complete meal

N.V.: Calories: 290, Fat: 9g, Carbs: 18g, Protein: 35g, Sugar: 5g

BAKED COD WITH MEDITERRANEAN TOMATO CONCASSE

P.T.: 20 min | **C.T.:** 20 min

M. of C.: Baking | **SERVES:** 4

INGR: 4 6-oz cod fillets

- 4 ripe tomatoes, finely chopped

- 1 C. Kalamata olives, pitted and sliced

- 2 cloves garlic, minced

- 1 Tbls capers, drained

- 2 Tbls extra virgin olive oil

- 1 Tbls balsamic vinegar

- 1 tsp dried oregano

- Fresh basil leaves, for garnish

- Salt and pepper to taste

PROC: Preheat oven to 375°F (190°C)

- In a bowl, combine tomatoes, olives, garlic, capers, olive oil, balsamic vinegar, oregano, salt, and pepper

- Place cod fillets in a baking dish and top with tomato mixture

- Bake for 20 min or until fish flakes easily with a fork

- Garnish with fresh basil before serving

TIPS: Serve with a side of sautéed spinach for added greens - Use cherry tomatoes for a sweeter concasse - Balsamic vinegar can be replaced with red wine vinegar for a different acidity level

N.V.: Calories: 310, Fat: 15g, Carbs: 10g, Protein: 35g, Sugar: 4g

BAKED COD WITH CAPER AND LEMON BUTTER SAUCE

P.T.: 10 min | **C.T.:** 15 min

M. of C.: Baking | **SERVES:** 4

INGR: 4 6-oz cod fillets

- 2 Tbls unsalted butter

- 1 Tbls lemon juice

- 1 tsp lemon zest

- 2 Tbls capers, drained

- 1 Tbls fresh dill, chopped

- Salt and pepper to taste

PROC: Preheat oven to 400°F (200°C)

- In a small saucepan, melt butter over medium heat

- Add lemon juice, zest, and capers to the butter and simmer for 2 min

- Season cod with salt and pepper and place in a baking dish

- Pour the lemon butter sauce over cod and sprinkle with dill

- Bake for 15 min or until cod is cooked through

TIPS: Lemon wedges on the side enhance the citrus flavor - Serve with roasted asparagus for a perfect pairing

N.V.: Calories: 220, Fat: 9g, Carbs: 2g, Protein: 35g, Sugar: 0g

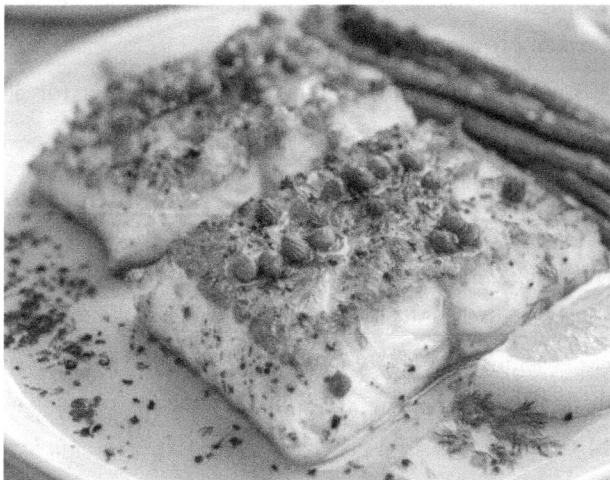

TURKEY CHILI

CLASSIC TURKEY CHILI

P.T.: 15 min. | **C.T.:** 45 min.

M. of C.: Stovetop | **SERVES:** 6

INGR: 2 lb. ground turkey

- 1 large yellow onion, diced

- 2 cloves garlic, minced

- 1 can (14.5 oz.) diced tomatoes

- 1 can (15 oz.) kidney beans, drained

- 1 can (8 oz.) tomato sauce

- 2 Tbls chili powder

- 1 Tbls ground cumin

- 1 tsp smoked paprika

- 1 tsp salt

- 1/2 tsp black pepper

- 2 C. chicken broth

- 1/4 C. fresh cilantro, chopped

- 1 Tbls olive oil

PROC: Heat the olive oil in a large pot over medium heat

- Add onions and garlic, sauté until translucent

- Add ground turkey, cook until browned

- Stir in chili powder, cumin, paprika, salt, and pepper

- Add diced tomatoes, kidney beans, tomato sauce, and chicken broth

- Bring to a boil, then reduce heat and simmer for 30 min.

- Stir in chopped cilantro before serving

TIPS: Serve with a dollop of Greek yogurt or a sprinkle of shredded cheddar cheese for extra flavor - Incorporate a side of cornbread to complement the chili's robust flavors - For a heartier meal, add a cup of diced bell peppers when sautéing the onions

N.V.: Calories: 320, Fat: 8g, Carbs: 19g, Protein: 35g, Sugar: 5g

TURKEY AND VEGGIE CHILI

P.T.: 20 min. | **C.T.:** 40 min.

M. of C.: Stovetop | **SERVES:** 5

INGR: 1.5 lb. ground turkey

- 1 red bell pepper, chopped

- 1 green bell pepper, chopped

- 1 zucchini, diced

- 1 yellow squash, diced

- 1 onion, chopped

- 2 carrots, peeled and chopped

- 3 Tbls tomato paste

- 1 can (15 oz.) black beans, drained

- 1 C. corn kernels, fresh or frozen

- 2 tsp chili powder

- 1 tsp cumin

- 3 C. vegetable broth

- 2 Tbls olive oil

- Salt and pepper to taste

PROC: Heat olive oil in a large saucepan over medium heat

- Add onion, red and green bell peppers, sauté until soft

- Add ground turkey, cook until no longer pink

- Stir in chili powder, cumin, and tomato paste

- Add zucchini, yellow squash, and carrots, cook for 5 min.

- Pour in vegetable broth, bring to a simmer

- Add black beans and corn, cook for another 15 min.

TIPS: Opt to garnish with avocado slices or a squeeze of lime for a fresh twist - Serve with a side of baked tortilla chips for added crunch

N.V.: Calories: 275, Fat: 10g, Carbs: 25g, Protein: 22g, Sugar: 7g

SPICY TURKEY AND SWEET POTATO CHILI

P.T.: 10 min. | **C.T.:** 50 min.

M. of C.: Stovetop | **SERVES:** 4

INGR: 1 lb. ground turkey

- 2 sweet potatoes, peeled and cubed

- 1 onion, diced

- 2 cloves garlic, minced

- 1 chipotle chili in adobo sauce, finely chopped

- 1 tsp ground cinnamon

- 1 tsp cayenne pepper

- 1 can (14.5 oz.) fire-roasted diced tomatoes

- 2 C. chicken stock

- 1 Tbls olive oil

- Salt and pepper to taste

PROC: Heat olive oil in a pot over medium heat

- Add onions and garlic, cook until they begin to soften

- Add ground turkey, breaking it up as it cooks until browned

- Stir in cinnamon, cayenne pepper, and chipotle chili

- Add sweet potatoes, fire-roasted tomatoes, and chicken stock

- Season with salt and pepper

- Bring to a simmer and cook until potatoes are tender, about 40 min.

TIPS: Top with fresh cilantro and a drizzle of sour cream for a creamy finish - Incorporate a sprinkle of toasted pumpkin seeds for crunch and added nutrition

- Pair with a rustic whole grain bread to soak up the hearty sauce

N.V.: Calories: 330, Fat: 9g, Carbs: 30g, Protein: 28g, Sugar: 8g

SPAGHETTI SQUASH WITH MARINARA AND MEATBALLS

SPAGHETTI SQUASH WITH MARINARA AND TURKEY MEATBALLS

P.T.: 20 min. | **C.T.:** 40 min.

M. of C.: Baking | **SERVES:** 4

INGR: 1 large spaghetti squash, halved lengthwise and seeded

- 1 lb. ground turkey

- 1 C. diced onions

- 1 Tbls. minced garlic

- 1 Tbls. Italian seasoning

- 1 egg

- ½ C. almond flour

- 2 C. marinara sauce

- 1 Tbls. olive oil

- Salt and pepper to taste

PROC: Preheat oven to 400°F (204°C)

- Brush squash halves with olive oil, season with salt and pepper, and place cut side down on baking sheet

- Roast in preheated oven for 40 min.

- While squash roasts, mix ground turkey, onions, garlic, Italian seasoning, egg, almond flour, salt, and pepper in a bowl

- Form into meatballs

- Heat olive oil in a skillet over medium heat, add meatballs, and cook until browned on all sides

- Add marinara sauce to pan, cover, and simmer until meatballs are cooked through

- Use a fork to shred squash into noodle-like strands

- Serve meatballs and sauce over spaghetti squash strands

TIPS: Add a sprinkle of fresh basil or parsley for garnish before serving - Use freshly grated Parmesan for added flavor

N.V.: Calories: 392, Fat: 22g, Carbs: 28g, Protein: 25g, Sugar: 14g

BRAISED SPAGHETTI SQUASH WITH CHERMOULA AND CRUMBLED FETA

P.T.: 15 min. | **C.T.:** 55 min.

M. of C.: Braising | **SERVES:** 4

INGR: 1 medium spaghetti squash

- 2 Tbls. olive oil

- 1 Tbls. Chermoula spice blend

- ½ C. vegetable broth

- 1 C. crumbled feta cheese

- Salt to taste

PROC: Preheat oven to 375°F (190°C)

- Halve squash and remove seeds

- Rub Chermoula spice blend and olive oil on the inside of squash

- Place cut side up in a baking dish

- Pour vegetable broth around the squash halves

- Cover with foil and bake for 45 min., or until tender

- Remove from oven, and use a fork to separate the squash strands

- Top with crumbled feta before serving

TIPS: Serve with an extra drizzle of olive oil if desired

- Pair with a side of sautéed greens for a complete meal

N.V.: Calories: 208, Fat: 15g, Carbs: 13g, Protein: 8g, Sugar: 6g

MISO GLAZED SPAGHETTI SQUASH WITH SESAME SEEDS

P.T.: 10 min. | **C.T.:** 50 min.

M. of C.: Roasting | **SERVES:** 4

INGR: 1 large spaghetti squash, halved and seeds removed

- 2 Tbls. miso paste

- 1 Tbls. honey

- 2 tsp. sesame oil

- 1 tsp. freshly grated ginger

- 1 Tbls. rice vinegar

- Sesame seeds for garnish

- Salt to taste

PROC: Preheat oven to 400°F (204°C)

- Mix together miso paste, honey, sesame oil, ginger, and rice vinegar to make glaze

- Brush the inside of squash halves with glaze

- Season with salt

- Place on lined baking sheet and roast for 50 min.

- Once cooked, use a fork to create spaghetti-like strands from the flesh

- Garnish with sesame seeds

TIPS: Make sure to evenly coat the squash with the miso glaze for optimum flavoring - Sprinkle toasted sesame seeds for added crunch and nuttiness

N.V.: Calories: 134, Fat: 4g, Carbs: 24g, Protein: 3g, Sugar: 10g

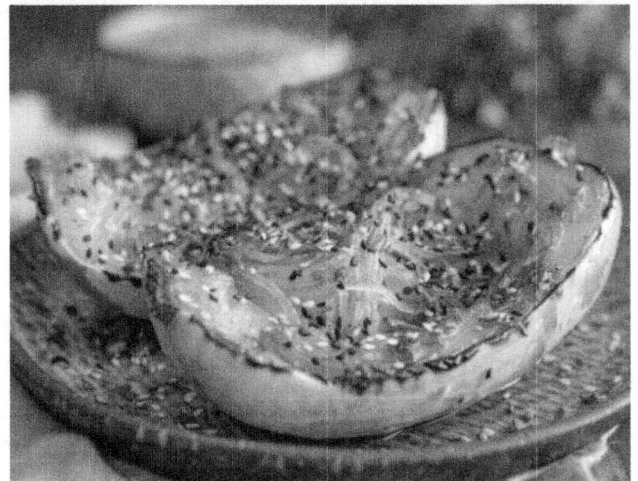

CHAPTER 10: SNACKS AND DESSERTS
1. HEALTHY SNACK IDEAS

We've all been there: those mid-afternoon slumps or post-dinner cravings that send us rummaging through the kitchen, seeking something that can satisfy without undoing the day's healthy choices. This pivotal moment can make or break your diet success, steering your carb cycling journey towards either a rewarding triumph or a guilt-ridden setback. It's here, in the humble choices of your daily snacking habits, that the foundation for sustainable weight management truly lies.

Healthy snacking, contrary to popular antics of dietary restriction, isn't about denying yourself the joys of eating. It's about smart, strategic eating that fuels your body while keeping your metabolic fire stoked. Imagine sitting down to a mid-morning snack – you reach for a crunchy, freshly-prepared veggie stick dipped in a rich, savory hummus. Not only does it crunch satisfyingly with each bite, but it also fills you up without weighing you down. Or, think about indulging in a cup of Greek yogurt, the creamy texture and sweet burst of berries mingling on your tongue, all while packing a potent protein punch that powers you through your next meeting or workout.

These aren't just temporary fillers; they are nutritional powerhouses that support your carb cycling method and bolster your energy throughout the day. By choosing snacks that are high in nutrients yet moderate in carbs and calories, you're better equipped to handle cravings, control portions at meals, and maintain a steady level of energy. It's all about keeping that delicate balance—aligning your carb intake with your daily activities and overall meal plan strategy.

By the end of this chapter, not only will you have a list of delicious, easy-to-prepare snacks that align with your carb cycling goals, but also you'll understand how these small bites fit into the larger puzzle of your dietary regimen. The right snack isn't just a treat; it's a tool—a delightful, enjoyable tool that keeps you on track without feeling deprived. Let's embark on transforming how you think about snacking, making it a purposeful and enjoyable part of your healthy lifestyle.

VEGGIE STICKS WITH HUMMUS

CLASSIC HUMMUS WITH RAINBOW VEGGIE STICKS

P.T.: 15 min. | **C.T.:** 0 min.
M. of C.: No Cooking | **SERVES:** 4
INGR: 1 C. canned chickpeas, rinsed and drained

- 2 Tbls tahini

- 1 garlic clove, minced

- Juice of 1 lemon

- 2 Tbls extra virgin olive oil

- 1/4 tsp ground cumin

- Salt and black pepper to taste

- Assorted veggie sticks (carrot, bell pepper, cucumber, celery)

PROC: Place chickpeas, tahini, garlic, lemon juice, olive oil, cumin, salt, and black pepper in a food processor and blend until smooth

- Adjust seasoning if necessary

- Serve with a variety of colorful veggie sticks

TIPS: Drizzle with a little extra olive oil and sprinkle with paprika before serving for added flavor and presentation - Keep the hummus refrigerated in an airtight container to maintain freshness - For extra zest, add a pinch of red pepper flakes
N.V.: Calories: 150, Fat: 10g, Carbs: 13g, Protein: 4g, Sugar: 2g

BEETROOT HUMMUS WITH SPICED VEGGIE STICKS

P.T.: 20 min. | **C.T.:** 0 min.

M. of C.: No Cooking | **SERVES:** 4

INGR: 1 C. cooked beetroot, chopped

- 1 C. canned chickpeas, rinsed and drained

- 1 Tbls tahini

- 2 garlic cloves, minced

- Juice of 1/2 lemon

- 3 Tbls extra virgin olive oil

- 1/4 tsp ground cumin

- Salt and black pepper to taste

- Dusting of ground coriander

- Veggie sticks (zucchini, yellow squash, snap peas, radishes)

PROC: Combine beetroot, chickpeas, tahini, garlic, lemon juice, olive oil, cumin, coriander, salt, and pepper in a food processor and process until creamy

- Serve chilled with an assortment of spiced veggie sticks

TIPS: Sprinkle hummus with sesame seeds for a crunch and visual appeal - Pinch of ground coriander can be added to the veggies as well before serving for an aromatic touch - Use a variety of unexpected vegetables like kohlrabi or jicama for the sticks to surprise and delight

N.V.: Calories: 135, Fat: 9g, Carbs: 12g, Protein: 3g, Sugar: 3g

AVOCADO LIME HUMMUS WITH HERBED VEGGIE STICKS

P.T.: 10 min. | **C.T.:** 0 min.

M. of C.: No Cooking | **SERVES:** 4

INGR: 1 ripe avocado, peeled and pitted

- 1 C. canned chickpeas, rinsed and drained

- 2 Tbls tahini

- 1 garlic clove, minced

- Juice of 1 lime

- 2 Tbls extra virgin olive oil

- Fresh cilantro, a handful, chopped

- Salt and chili flakes to taste

- Veggie sticks (asparagus, green beans, baby carrots, cherry tomatoes)

PROC: In a blender, combine avocado, chickpeas, tahini, garlic, lime juice, olive oil, cilantro, salt, and chili flakes until smooth

- Serve immediately with herbed veggie sticks, using fresh cilantro and chili flakes to season the vegetables

TIPS: Garnish hummus with a lime wedge for a burst of freshness - Keep hummus vibrant green by adding a touch of lime zest to the blend - Explore using blanched vegetables like asparagus and green beans for dipping to add a delightful crunch

N.V.: Calories: 165, Fat: 12g, Carbs: 14g, Protein: 4g, Sugar: 2g

GREEK YOGURT AND BERRY CUPS

VANILLA CHAI GREEK YOGURT PARFAITS

P.T.: 10 min | **C.T.:** 0 min

M. of C.: No Cooking | **SERVES:** 4

INGR: 2 C. Greek yogurt, plain

- 1 Tbls chai spice mix

- 2 Tbls honey

- 1 C. granola, preferably no added sugar

- 1 C. mixed berries (blueberries, raspberries, strawberries), fresh or thawed

- 1 Tbls chia seeds

PROC: Combine Greek yogurt with chai spice mix and honey in a mixing bowl

- In glass cups, layer the mixed berries, then a layer of the spiced Greek yogurt, followed by a sprinkling of granola

- Repeat layering until the cups are filled, finishing with a layer of berries topped with chia seeds

TIPS: Serve immediately or chill in the refrigerator for a richer infusion of chai flavors - Customize by using different types of berries or adding a pinch of cinnamon on top for extra zest

N.V.: Calories: 240, Fat: 6g, Carbs: 34g, Protein: 13g, Sugar: 18g

PISTACHIO AND MATCHA GREEK YOGURT DELIGHT

P.T.: 15 min | **C.T.:** 0 min

M. of C.: No Cooking | **SERVES:** 2

INGR: 1½ C. Greek yogurt, plain

- 2 tsp matcha powder

- 1 Tbls honey

- ¼ C. pistachios, shelled and chopped

- 1 tsp lemon zest

- ½ C. kiwi, peeled and sliced

PROC: Stir matcha powder and honey into the Greek yogurt until well blended

- Divide the flavored yogurt into serving bowls

- Garnish each serving with sliced kiwi, chopped pistachios, and a sprinkle of lemon zest

TIPS: Enhance the dish by drizzling a little extra honey over the top if a sweeter taste is preferred - For a crunchier texture, add more pistachios or consider a sprinkle of flax seeds

N.V.: Calories: 215, Fat: 8g, Carbs: 24g, Protein: 15g, Sugar: 16g

BERRY LAVENDER GREEK YOGURT CUPS

P.T.: 12 min | **C.T.:** 0 min

M. of C.: No Cooking | **SERVES:** 3

INGR: 1½ C. Greek yogurt, plain

- 1 Tbls dried lavender buds, crushed

- 1 Tbls honey

- ½ C. blueberries

- ½ C. raspberries

- 1 Tbls almond slivers

- Fresh mint leaves for garnish

PROC: Infuse the Greek yogurt with crushed lavender buds and honey, mixing thoroughly

- In decorative cups, arrange a base of fresh blueberries and raspberries

- Spoon the lavender-infused yogurt over the berries

- Garnish with almond slivers and mint leaves

TIPS: For a more intense lavender flavor, allow the yogurt to infuse overnight in the refrigerator - Decorate with additional berries or edible flowers for a more visually appealing presentation

N.V.: Calories: 180, Fat: 5g, Carbs: 21g, Protein: 14g, Sugar: 15g

MIXED NUTS AND SEEDS

SAVORY ROSEMARY NUT MIX

P.T.: 15 min | **C.T.:** 20 min

M. of C.: Baking | **SERVES:** 6

INGR: 1 C. raw cashews

- 1 C. raw almonds

- 1 C. walnuts

- 1 Tbls fresh rosemary, finely chopped

- 2 Tbls olive oil

- 1 tsp smoked paprika

- 1/2 tsp sea salt

- 1/4 tsp garlic powder

PROC: Preheat oven to 350°F (175°C)

- Combine nuts, rosemary, olive oil, smoked paprika, sea salt, and garlic powder in a large bowl and stir until nuts are evenly coated

- Spread the nut mixture on a baking sheet lined with parchment paper

- Bake in preheated oven until nuts are golden and fragrant, about 20 min, stirring halfway through

TIPS: Store in an airtight container to maintain freshness and crispness - Serve as a standalone snack or as a topping for salads

N.V.: Calories: 285, Fat: 24g, Carbs: 12g, Protein: 8g, Sugar: 2g

MAPLE CINNAMON SEED CRUNCH

P.T.: 10 min | **C.T.:** 15 min

M. of C.: Baking | **SERVES:** 4

INGR: 1/2 C. pumpkin seeds

- 1/2 C. sunflower seeds

- 1/4 C. sesame seeds

- 2 Tbls maple syrup

- 1 tsp ground cinnamon

- A pinch of salt

PROC: Preheat oven to 325°F (163°C)

- Mix all seeds together with maple syrup, cinnamon, and salt in a bowl until well coated

- Spread the seed mixture evenly onto a lined baking sheet

- Bake for about 15 min or until seeds are toasted and the syrup has caramelized, stirring occasionally

TIPS: Cool completely before breaking into clusters - Adds a sweet crunch to morning yogurt or oatmeal

N.V.: Calories: 180, Fat: 14g, Carbs: 8g, Protein: 6g, Sugar: 4g

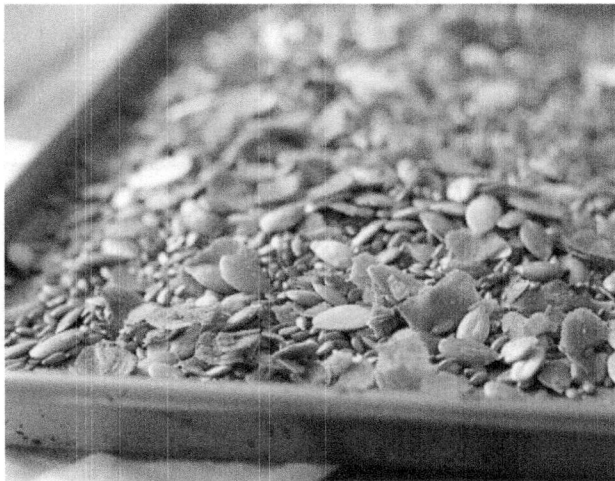

SPICY TAMARI TRAIL MIX

P.T.: 8 min | **C.T.:** 0 min

M. of C.: No Cooking | **SERVES:** 8

INGR: 1 C. pecans

- 1 C. dried cranberries

- 1 C. roasted chickpeas

- 1/2 C. raw pistachios

- 3 Tbls tamari sauce

- 1 tsp chili powder

- 1/2 tsp ground cumin

PROC: In a large bowl, toss the pecans, cranberries, chickpeas, pistachios, tamari sauce, chili powder, and cumin until everything is evenly coated

- Let the mixture sit for about 5 min to absorb flavors

- Spread out on parchment paper to dry slightly if wet

TIPS: Can be portioned into individual snack bags for a quick grab-and-go option - The unique blend of spicy and umami flavors makes this an exciting alternative to traditional trail mixes

N.V.: Calories: 210, Fat: 15g, Carbs: 18g, Protein: 6g, Sugar: 11g

2. LOW-CARB DESSERTS

Imagine settling into the evening with a satisfying dessert that doesn't derail your low-carb goals but instead embraces them. It's possible, and this chapter is dedicated to transforming the notion that desserts are merely indulgent treats into a reality where they can be both delightful and conducive to your health objectives.

In the realm of low-carb eating, desserts are not just afterthoughts; they are testament to flexibility and creativity in the kitchen. You might wonder, can something as traditionally decadent as desserts be friendly to a low-carb lifestyle? Absolutely, and the secret lies in selecting the right ingredients and embracing natural, low-carb sweeteners such as stevia, erythritol, or monk fruit which offer the sweetness we crave, without the carbohydrate load that we aim to avoid. Take, for instance, the transformation of a classic chocolate cake into a keto-friendly delight using almond flour and cocoa powder, which not only cuts down the carbs but also increases the nutritional value with a higher protein content. Or consider a berry cheesecake where the base is crafted from ground nuts rather than biscuits, slashing the carbs while enhancing the fiber and healthy fats.

The beauty of these desserts goes beyond their carb count. Each recipe is an opportunity to experiment with flavors and textures, to indulge in the culinary artistry of creating something truly spectacular that supports your dietary goals. These aren't just treats; they're strategic, tasty components of your carb cycling plan, designed to keep you satisfied and on track.

Each dessert recipe in this chapter will guide you through the process, ensuring what ends up on your plate supports your wellness journey. Whether you are rounding off a dinner or seeking a mid-afternoon pick-me-up, these low-carb desserts provide a guilt-free way to enjoy the sweeter side of life. So, let's turn the page and start exploring the delicious possibilities that await.

KETO CHOCOLATE MUG CAKE

KETO CHOCOLATE MUG CAKE

P.T.: 5 min | **C.T.:** 1 min
M. of C.: Microwave | **SERVES:** 1
INGR: 4 Tbls almond flour

- 1 Tbls cocoa powder, unsweetened

- 1/4 tsp baking powder

- 1 Tbls erythritol

- 1 large egg

- 2 Tbls heavy cream

- 1/2 tsp vanilla extract

- 1 Tbls unsalted butter, melted

- Pinch of salt

PROC: Combine almond flour, cocoa powder, baking powder, erythritol, and salt in a microwave-safe mug

- Add egg, heavy cream, vanilla extract, and melted butter to the dry ingredients

- Mix thoroughly until smooth

- Microwave on high for 60 seconds

TIPS: Check doneness with a toothpick - if it comes out clean, it's ready - If you prefer a moister cake, reduce the cooking time by a few seconds - Serve with a dollop of sugar-free whipped cream or a sprinkle of keto-friendly chocolate chips

N.V.: Calories: 410, Fat: 36g, Carbs: 8g, Protein: 12g, Sugar: 1g

CINNAMON SWIRL KETO MUG CAKE

P.T.: 6 min | **C.T.:** 1 min
M. of C.: Microwave | **SERVES:** 1
INGR: 3 Tbls coconut flour

- 1/2 tsp cinnamon

- 1/4 tsp nutmeg

- 1 Tbls erythritol plus extra for sprinkling

- 1/4 tsp baking powder

- 1 large egg

- 1 Tbls heavy cream

- 1 tsp vanilla extract

- 1 Tbls coconut oil, melted

PROC: Mix coconut flour, cinnamon, nutmeg, erythritol, and baking powder in a mug

- Add egg, heavy cream, vanilla extract, and melted coconut oil

- Stir until you achieve a uniform batter

- Sprinkle additional erythritol on top for a 'sugar crust' effect

- Microwave on high for about 70 seconds

TIPS: Serve immediately for best texture - Can be enjoyed with a side of keto vanilla ice cream for a decadent dessert - Add a touch of unsweetened apple sauce for extra moisture without significant carb increase

N.V.: Calories: 320, Fat: 28g, Carbs: 9g, Protein: 7g, Sugar: 2g

KETO LEMON POPPY SEED MUG CAKE

P.T.: 7 min | **C.T.:** 1 min
M. of C.: Microwave | **SERVES:** 1
INGR: 3 Tbls almond flour

- 1 Tbls coconut flour

- 1/2 tsp baking powder

- 1 Tbls erythritol

- 1 Tbls poppy seeds

- Zest of 1 lemon

- 1 large egg

- 1 Tbls lemon juice

- 2 Tbls unsalted butter, melted

- 1 Tbls unsweetened almond milk

PROC: In a mug, blend almond flour, coconut flour, baking powder, erythritol, and poppy seeds

- Add lemon zest, egg, lemon juice, melted butter, and almond milk to the dry mix

- Whisk until the batter is smooth

- Microwave for about 70 seconds

TIPS: Let it rest for a couple of minutes after microwaving to develop flavors - Garnish with a slice of lemon or a light drizzle of keto-friendly lemon glaze for extra zest - Adjust sweetness by increasing or reducing erythritol according to taste

N.V.: Calories: 375, Fat: 34g, Carbs: 7g, Protein: 9g, Sugar: 1g

ALMOND FLOUR COOKIES

CLASSIC ALMOND FLOUR COOKIES

P.T.: 15 min. | **C.T.:** 12 min.
M. of C.: Baking | **SERVES:** 24
INGR: 2 C. almond flour

- 1/3 C. granulated erythritol

- 1 large egg

- 1/4 C. unsalted butter, softened

- 1 tsp. vanilla extract

- 1/2 tsp. baking soda

- 1/4 tsp. sea salt

PROC: Preheat oven to 350°F (175°C)

- In a bowl, cream together butter and erythritol until fluffy

- Beat in vanilla extract and egg

- In a separate bowl, whisk almond flour, baking soda, and sea salt

- Gradually combine dry ingredients into wet ingredients until dough forms

- Roll dough into 1-inch balls and place on parchment-lined baking sheet

- Press down lightly to flatten

- Bake until edges are golden, about 12 min.

TIPS: Chill dough for 30 min. before baking to enhance flavors - Flatten cookies with a fork for a textured look

N.V.: Calories: 80, Fat: 7g, Carbs: 2g, Protein: 3g, Sugar: 1g

LAVENDER ALMOND SHORTBREAD

P.T.: 20 min. | **C.T.:** 15 min.
M. of C.: Baking | **SERVES:** 18
INGR: 2 C. almond flour

- 1/2 C. coconut oil, solid

- 1/4 C. honey

- 2 Tbls. culinary lavender flowers, finely chopped

- 1 tsp. lemon zest

PROC: Preheat oven to 325°F (163°C)

- Combine almond flour, lavender, and lemon zest in a bowl

- In another bowl, blend coconut oil and honey until smooth

- Mix dry and wet ingredients to form a crumbly dough

- Press dough into an ungreased square baking pan

- Score into squares with a knife

- Bake until edges are light golden, about 15 min.

TIPS: Use food processor for finer lavender texture - Cool in pan before slicing to prevent crumbling
N.V.: Calories: 90, Fat: 8g, Carbs: 4g, Protein: 2g, Sugar: 3g

SPICED ALMOND COOKIES

P.T.: 12 min. | **C.T.:** 10 min.
M. of C.: Baking | **SERVES:** 20
INGR: 1.5 C. almond flour

- 1/4 C. coconut sugar

- 1 tsp. ground cinnamon

- 1/2 tsp. ground nutmeg

- 1/4 tsp. ground ginger

- 1 large egg

- 1/4 C. unsalted butter, melted

- 1 tsp. almond extract

PROC: Preheat oven to 375°F (190°C)

- Whisk together almond flour, cinnamon, nutmeg, and ginger in a bowl

- In another bowl, mix melted butter, coconut sugar, almond extract, and egg until smooth

- Combine wet and dry ingredients to make cookie dough

- Spoon dough onto a prepared baking sheet

- Bake until edges are just browned, about 10 min.

TIPS: Allow cookies to cool on the tray for 5 min. before transferring to a wire rack - Experiment with adding clove for extra warmth
N.V.: Calories: 70, Fat: 6g, Carbs: 3g, Protein: 2g, Sugar: 2g

BERRY CHEESECAKE BITES

RASPBERRY ALMOND CHEESECAKE BITES

P.T.: 20 min | **C.T.:** 15 min
M. of C.: Baking | **SERVES:** 24
INGR: 1 C. almond flour

- ¼ C. coconut flour

- ⅓ C. erythritol

- 6 Tbls unsalted butter, melted

- 1 tsp vanilla extract

- 8 oz. cream cheese, softened

- ½ C. sour cream

- 1 large egg

- ¼ C. erythritol

- ½ tsp almond extract

- ½ C. fresh raspberries

PROC: Combine almond flour, coconut flour, ⅓ cup erythritol, melted butter, and vanilla extract in a bowl

- Press mixture into the bottom of mini muffin tins to form crusts

- Bake the crusts at 350°F (175°C) for 5 min

- Mix cream cheese, sour cream, egg, ¼ cup erythritol, and almond extract until smooth

- Spoon cream cheese mixture over crusts

- Press a raspberry into the center of each bite

- Bake for an additional 10 min or until set

TIPS: Chill in the fridge before serving to enhance firmness - Use a silicone mini muffin pan for easier removal

N.V.: Calories: 120, Fat: 10g, Carbs: 3g, Protein: 2g, Sugar: 2g

LIME & BLUEBERRY CHEESECAKE BITES

P.T.: 25 min | **C.T.:** 20 min
M. of C.: Baking | **SERVES:** 18
INGR: 1 C. crushed pecans

- 1 Tbls melted coconut oil

- 1 tsp stevia

- 8 oz. cream cheese, softened

- ¼ C. Greek yogurt

- 1 large egg

- 2 Tbls lime juice

- Zest of 1 lime

- ¼ C. stevia

- ⅓ C. fresh blueberries

PROC: Blend crushed pecans, coconut oil, and 1 tsp stevia to form a coarse crust mixture

- Press this into mini tart pans

- Bake at 350°F (175°C) for 7 min

- Combine cream cheese, Greek yogurt, egg, lime juice, lime zest, and ¼ C. stevia until creamy

- Fill tart shells with mixture and top each with blueberries

- Bake for 13 min until slightly golden

TIPS: Allow to cool to room temperature then refrigerate for 2 hrs before serving - Garnish with extra lime zest for a zesty kick

N.V.: Calories: 135, Fat: 11g, Carbs: 4g, Protein: 3g, Sugar: 2g

COCONUT MATCHA CHEESECAKE BITES

P.T.: 15 min | **C.T.:** 18 min
M. of C.: Baking | **SERVES:** 20
INGR: 1 C. shredded coconut, unsweetened

- ¼ C. coconut oil, melted

- 1 Tbls monk fruit sweetener

- 8 oz. cream cheese, softened

- ¼ C. coconut cream

- 1 large egg

- 1 Tbls matcha powder

- ¼ C. monk fruit sweetener

PROC: Mix shredded coconut, melted coconut oil, and 1 Tbls monk fruit sweetener; press into the bottoms of a lined mini muffin tray

- Bake at 350°F (175°C) for 6 min

- Combine cream cheese, coconut cream, egg, matcha powder, and ¼ C. monk fruit sweetener until smooth

- Spoon over baked coconut bases

- Bake for additional 12 min or until filling is set

TIPS: Refrigerate overnight to firm up the bites - Top with a sprinkle of shredded coconut or drizzle with melted dark chocolate for extra indulgence

N.V.: Calories: 98, Fat: 9g, Carbs: 3g, Protein: 2g, Sugar: 1g

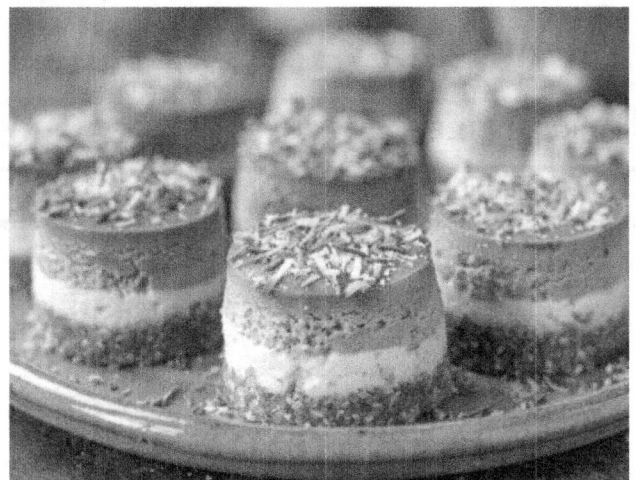

3. HIGH-CARB DESSERTS

Indulging in desserts can often feel like a delightful rebellion against the usual strictures of dieting, especially when you are working hard to manage your carbohydrate intake. But what if I told you that these sweet indulgences could be part of your balanced carb cycling plan? Yes, it's true—welcome to the world of high-carb desserts that align perfectly with your high-carb days!

Imagine this: It's been an energetic day; you adhered to your meal plan, fueled your body well, and now, it's time for a reward. Not just any reward, but a delicious, comforting, and satisfying dessert that doesn't derail your progress. This doesn't have to be a daydream. High-carb desserts are crafted not only to satisfy your sweet tooth but also to support your dietary goals, replenishing glycogen stores after intensive activities or workouts, making them as beneficial as they are delightful.

Think of scrumptious baked apples, warm and spiced with cinnamon, or a dense, chewy oatmeal raisin cookie. These aren't just treats; they're tools. While they bring a sense of indulgence, these desserts are carefully designed to fit into a well-structured eating plan, giving you energy when your body needs it most—on those high-carb days meant to refuel and recharge.

Crafting these desserts takes into account not just their carbohydrate content but the textures and flavors that evoke comfort and joy. A fruit sorbet, light and refreshing, or a rich, fruity smoothie bowl can be just the uplifting finish to a day's meal plan. These recipes show that a nutritional approach focusing on weight management can indeed embrace the sweeter things in life without guilt.

In this section of the book, I'll guide you through integrating these delectable desserts into your high-carb days, maintaining the balance that your diet demands. It's all about the strategic placement of carbs, and what better way to enjoy them than through desserts that uplift your spirit and aid in your fitness and health goals? Here's to enjoying every bite, guilt-free!

BAKED APPLES WITH CINNAMON

CHAI-SPICED BAKED APPLES

P.T.: 15 min. | **C.T.:** 45 min.

M. of C.: Baking | **SERVES:** 4

INGR: 4 large firm apples (e.g., Honeycrisp or Fuji)

- 1 C. rolled oats

- 4 Tbls. honey

- 2 Tbls. unsalted butter, melted

- 1 tsp. ground cinnamon

- 1/2 tsp. ground cardamom

- 1/4 tsp. ground nutmeg

- 1/4 tsp. ground cloves

- 1/4 tsp. ground ginger

- 2 C. apple cider

PROC: Core apples and hollow out, leaving a thick border intact

- Mix oats, honey, melted butter, cinnamon, cardamom, nutmeg, cloves, and ginger in a bowl

- Stuff mixture into hollowed apples

- Place apples in a baking dish and pour apple cider around them

- Bake in preheated oven at 375°F (190°C) until apples are soft and stuffing is golden brown

TIPS: Serve with a dollop of Greek yogurt for added creaminess - Pair with a warm cup of chai tea for enhanced flavors

N.V.: Calories: 295, Fat: 7g, Carbs: 58g, Protein: 3g, Sugar: 44g

MAPLE GLAZED BAKED APPLES WITH WALNUTS

P.T.: 10 min. | **C.T.:** 30 min.

M. of C.: Baking | **SERVES:** 4

INGR: 4 Granny Smith apples

- 1/4 C. walnuts, chopped

- 4 Tbls. pure maple syrup

- 1 Tbls. dark brown sugar

- 2 Tbls. unsalted butter

- 1/2 tsp. vanilla extract

- 1/2 tsp. ground cinnamon

PROC: Core and slice apples into half-inch rings, removing seeds

- Arrange apple slices in a single layer on a baking sheet

- Mix maple syrup, brown sugar, butter, vanilla extract, and cinnamon in a saucepan and heat until bubbling

- Drizzle glaze over apple slices and sprinkle with chopped walnuts

- Bake at 400°F (204°C) until apples are tender

TIPS: Great served with vanilla ice cream or as a topping for pancakes - Can be stored in an airtight container in the fridge for up to three days

N.V.: Calories: 210, Fat: 9g, Carbs: 34g, Protein: 2g, Sugar: 27g

CIDER-POACHED BAKED APPLES WITH STAR ANISE

P.T.: 20 min. | **C.T.:** 40 min.

M. of C.: Baking | **SERVES:** 4

INGR: 4 large apples

- 1 C. apple cider

- 2 star anise

- 4 Tbls. golden raisins

- 2 cinnamon sticks

- 2 Tbls. dark rum

- 1 Tbls. brown sugar

- Zest of 1 orange

PROC: Core apples and score around the midpoint to prevent splitting

- Place each apple on a small square of foil

- Mix apple cider, star anise, raisins, rum, and brown sugar in a bowl

- Pour mixture into apple cavities and over them, adding a cinnamon stick to each foil square

- Enclose apples in foil and bake at 350°F (177°C) until tender

TIPS: Can be enjoyed hot or cold - Perfect for festive occasions or as a cozy dessert

N.V.: Calories: 190, Fat: 0.5g, Carbs: 49g, Protein: 1g, Sugar: 38g

OATMEAL RAISIN COOKIES

CLASSIC CHEWY OATMEAL RAISIN COOKIES

P.T.: 15 min | **C.T.:** 12 min

M. of C.: Baking | **SERVES:** 24

INGR: 1¾ C. all-purpose flour

- ½ tsp baking soda

- ¼ tsp salt

- ¾ C. unsalted butter, softened

- 1 ¼ C. brown sugar, packed

- ¼ C. granulated sugar

- 2 eggs

- 2 tsp vanilla extract

- 3 C. old-fashioned oats

- 1 C. raisins

- 1 tsp cinnamon powder

PROC: Preheat oven to 375°F (190°C)

- Whisk together flour, baking soda, salt, and cinnamon in a bowl

- In a separate bowl, cream the butter with both sugars using an electric mixer until light and fluffy

- Beat in eggs one at a time, then add vanilla extract

- Gradually fold in the flour mixture until just combined

- Stir in oats and raisins

- Drop rounded tablespoonfuls onto baking sheets lined with parchment paper, spacing them 2 inches apart

- Bake until edges are golden, about 12 minutes

TIPS: Allow cookies to cool on the baking sheet for 5 minutes before transferring to a wire rack to cool completely - Keep cookies in an airtight container to maintain freshness - For a nuttier flavor, add ½ C. chopped walnuts or pecans to the dough

N.V.: Calories: 190, Fat: 7g, Carbs: 29g, Protein: 3g, Sugar: 13g

SPICED ORANGE OATMEAL COOKIES

P.T.: 20 min | **C.T.:** 14 min

M. of C.: Baking | **SERVES:** 20

INGR: 1½ C. whole wheat flour

- 1 tsp ground ginger

- ½ tsp nutmeg

- ½ tsp clove

- 1 orange, zested and juiced

- ½ C. coconut oil, melted

- 1 C. coconut sugar

- 2 eggs

- 1 tsp vanilla extract

- 2½ C. rolled oats

- 1 C. golden raisins

PROC: Preheat oven to 350°F (175°C)

- Combine flour, ginger, nutmeg, clove, and orange zest in a bowl

- In another bowl, mix coconut oil, coconut sugar, and half of the orange juice until well blended

- Beat in eggs and vanilla extract

- Add dry ingredients to wet ingredients and mix until incorporated

- Stir in oats and golden raisins

- Spoon cookie dough by Tbls onto baking sheets lined with parchment

- Bake until cookies are just firm and lightly browned on the edges, about 14 minutes

TIPS: Sprinkle warm cookies with a little extra coconut sugar and a drizzle of the remaining orange juice for added zest - Store cookies in a cool, dry place to prolong freshness - Experiment with adding chopped dried figs instead of raisins for a different flavor

N.V.: Calories: 175, Fat: 8g, Carbs: 25g, Protein: 3g, Sugar: 10g

TROPICAL TWIST OATMEAL COOKIES

P.T.: 18 min | **C.T.:** 10 min

M. of C.: Baking | **SERVES:** 18

INGR: 1 C. spelt flour

- 1 tsp baking powder

- ¼ tsp sea salt

- ½ C. raw cane sugar

- ½ C. unsalted butter, room temperature

- 1 egg

- 1 tsp almond extract

- 2 C. quick-cooking oats

- ⅔ C. shredded coconut

- ½ C. dried pineapple, chopped

- ½ C. macadamia nuts, chopped

PROC: Preheat oven to 375°F (190°C)

- Mix spelt flour, baking powder, and salt in a small bowl

- In a larger bowl, cream butter and cane sugar until fluffy

- Add egg and almond extract, mix well

- Gradually incorporate the dry ingredients until combined

- Fold in oats, coconut, pineapple, and macadamia nuts

- Drop spoonfuls of dough onto prepared cookie sheets

- Bake until the edges begin to brown, around 10 minutes

TIPS: Cool cookies on the sheet for two minutes before removing to a cooling rack - Mixing in a tablespoon of rum with the wet ingredients can enhance the tropical flavors - Press a small piece of additional dried pineapple on top of each cookie before baking for a decorative touch

N.V.: Calories: 160, Fat: 8g, Carbs: 21g, Protein: 2g, Sugar: 9g

FRUIT SORBET

MANGO LIME SORBET

P.T.: 15 min | **C.T.:** 0 min

M. of C.: Freezing | **SERVES:** 4

INGR: 2 C. mango, peeled and cubed

- Juice of 2 limes

- 1 Tbls honey

- 1 tsp fresh mint, finely chopped

- 1/4 C. water

PROC: Puree mango, lime juice, honey, mint, and water in a blender until smooth

- Pour mixture into a shallow baking dish

- Freeze for at least 4 hrs, scraping with a fork every hour to break up ice crystals

TIPS: Serve immediately for the best flavor and texture

- If sorbet is too hard, let sit at room temperature for a few minutes before serving - Top with extra mint leaves for a refreshing twist

N.V.: Calories: 110, Fat: 0g, Carbs: 28g, Protein: 1g, Sugar: 24g

RASPBERRY PEACH SORBET

P.T.: 20 min | **C.T.:** 0 min

M. of C.: Freezing | **SERVES:** 4

INGR: 3 C. raspberries

- 2 peaches, peeled and diced

- Juice of 1 lemon

- 1 Tbls agave syrup

PROC: Combine raspberries, peaches, lemon juice, and agave in a food processor and blend until smooth

- Strain through a fine mesh sieve to remove raspberry seeds

- Transfer to a freezing container and freeze until solid, about 5 hr

TIPS: Mash with a fork before serving to create a fluffy texture - Pair with a sprig of mint or basil for a gourmet touch

N.V.: Calories: 90, Fat: 0.5g, Carbs: 22g, Protein: 1g, Sugar: 20g

KIWI STRAWBERRY SORBET

P.T.: 10 min | **C.T.:** 0 min

M. of C.: Freezing | **SERVES:** 4

INGR: 1 pt. strawberries, hulled

- 4 kiwis, peeled and sliced

- Juice of 1 orange

- 2 Tbls honey

PROC: Blend strawberries, kiwis, orange juice, and honey in a food processor until smooth

- Pour into an ice cream maker and churn according to manufacturer's instructions, about 20-30 min

- Transfer to a container and freeze until firm

TIPS: Serve in chilled bowls for an extra cool sensation

- Garnish with slices of fresh kiwi or strawberry to enhance the visual appeal - Drizzle a little extra honey on top before serving for added sweetness

N.V.: Calories: 120, Fat: 0.5g, Carbs: 30g, Protein: 1g, Sugar: 25g

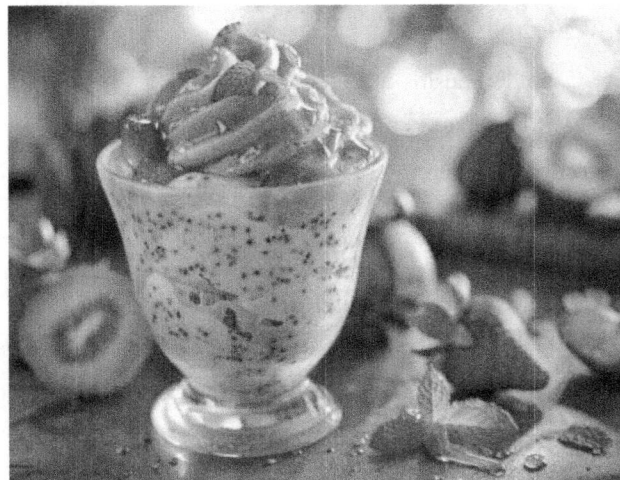

CHAPTER 11: TIPS FOR LONG-TERM SUCCESS

As we close on this transformative journey with "The New Carb Cycling System," you may find yourself at the threshold of what feels like a conclusive phase. Embrace this new beginning rather than viewing it as the end of a strictly outlined program. Chapter 11 is designed not just to congratulate you on your commitments thus far but to smoothly transition you from a structured system to an adaptable, enduring lifestyle.

Imagine your journey through this book as the planting of a garden. Initially, we meticulously outlined where to place each seed and how to care for them—watering, sunlight, nutrient administration—all under careful scrutiny. You've done the work, watched the first sprouts appear, and perhaps enjoyed a few homegrown meals. Now, as any seasoned gardener would tell you, the real task begins in nurturing this garden to thrive year after year, through changing seasons and varying climates.

This chapter imparts wisdom for long-term cultivation of your health and fitness routine. It's about recognizing that the lifestyle you've structured around carb cycling need not be rigid. Life will throw unforeseen challenges your way—special family dinners, urgent work deadlines, or simply a craving that doesn't fit the day's macros. Here, we'll explore how to adapt the principles you've learned, flexing them to fit life's ebbs and flows without losing sight of your overarching goals.

Moreover, this is about crafting sustainability through community, intentionality, and a mindset focused on progress rather than perfection. Emphasis will be placed on how to adjust your meals and exercise routines, sure, but also on fostering relationships with those who support your goals, whether they're family members, friends, or part of broader health-oriented communities.

Your path to sustained health is inherently personal and ever-evolving. Let this chapter serve as a guide to maintaining your results, adapting your meal plans, and embracing an empowered, healthy lifestyle that lasts a lifetime. Cheers to your continued success, with every mindful bite and every step forward.

1. MAINTAINING YOUR RESULTS

Maintaining your results is the ultimate goal of any weight loss journey, and it's the part that requires the most vigilance and adaptability. You've done the hard work to shed the pounds, balance your diet, and establish a routine that works for you. Now, the challenge is to keep the momentum going and avoid slipping back into old habits. The good news is that by integrating a few key strategies into your daily life, you can ensure that your hard-earned progress is not only maintained but also becomes second nature.

Strategies for Staying on Track

Staying on track is less about perfection and more about consistency. Life will always throw curveballs, whether it's a hectic work schedule, social gatherings, or just a craving that seems too tempting to resist. The key is to navigate these situations with a plan and a mindset that's focused on the long-term benefits of your efforts.

First, it's crucial to keep your goals front and center. Remind yourself regularly why you embarked on this journey in the first place. Whether it was to improve your health, boost your energy levels, or feel more confident in your own skin, these motivations are your anchor. Create a vision board, set reminders on your phone, or keep a journal where you reflect on your progress and future aspirations. These simple acts help keep your commitment alive, even on tough days. Another vital strategy is to continue monitoring your progress. This doesn't mean obsessing over the scale; instead, focus on how your clothes fit, how you feel throughout the day, and how your energy levels fluctuate. Regularly checking in with yourself allows you to make minor adjustments before any backsliding becomes significant. Keep a food journal or use a tracking app to log your meals and workouts. This practice not only keeps you accountable but also helps you identify patterns that may need tweaking.

Finally, embrace flexibility without losing sight of your goals. The rigidity that might have been necessary during the initial phase of your journey isn't sustainable long-term. Instead, learn to be adaptable. If you know you have a busy week ahead, prepare meals in advance or opt for quick, healthy options that require minimal preparation. If a special occasion arises, enjoy it without guilt, and simply get back on track with your next meal. Flexibility is about making the healthiest choice possible in any given situation, not about being perfect.

Adapting the Meal Plans for Maintenance

As you transition from weight loss to maintenance, your dietary needs will shift slightly. The goal now is to maintain your current weight, which may require adjusting your calorie intake and macronutrient distribution. However, this doesn't mean abandoning the strategies that got you here. Instead, it's about fine-tuning them to suit your new goals.

One of the first steps is to assess your caloric needs. As you lose weight, your body requires fewer calories to maintain its current state. This is a normal part of the process, and it's important to avoid frustration if your progress slows. Use an online calculator or consult with a nutritionist to determine your new maintenance calorie level. From there, you can make small adjustments to your meal plans, such as slightly increasing your portion sizes or incorporating more healthy fats, which are more calorie-dense.

Next, consider the variety in your diet. While it's easy to stick to the meals you've come to love, introducing new recipes and ingredients can keep things interesting and prevent boredom. Experiment with different cuisines, seasonal produce, and cooking methods to discover new favorites. This approach not only makes meal planning more enjoyable but also ensures that you're getting a wide range of nutrients.

Another key aspect of maintenance is listening to your body's hunger and fullness cues. During the weight loss phase, you might have been more focused on portion control and meal timing. Now, it's about tuning into your body's signals and eating when you're truly hungry, rather than out of habit or boredom. This intuitive approach to eating helps prevent overeating and promotes a healthier relationship with food.

Meal planning should also remain a priority. Even though you're in maintenance mode, planning your meals ahead of time can prevent impulsive decisions that could derail your progress. Continue batch cooking, keeping healthy snacks on hand, and planning your meals around your schedule. By staying organized, you make it easier to stick to your goals.

Keeping Up with Exercise

Exercise plays a crucial role in maintaining your weight and overall health. The routines you've established during your weight loss phase should continue, but with an eye towards sustainability and enjoyment. Exercise shouldn't feel like a chore; it should be something you look forward to as a part of your daily life.

First, re-evaluate your workout routine. As your fitness level improves, your body adapts to the exercises you're doing. This means that over time, you might burn fewer calories doing the same activities. To combat this, consider increasing the intensity of your workouts or incorporating new types of exercise. This could be as simple as adding an extra day of cardio, trying a new fitness class, or incorporating more resistance training. Variety not only keeps your body challenged but also prevents burnout.

Secondly, find activities you enjoy. The best exercise is the one you'll stick with long-term. If you dread going to the gym, explore other options like hiking, swimming, dancing, or even joining a recreational sports league. The more you enjoy your workouts, the more likely you are to stay consistent. Remember, exercise is not just about burning calories; it's also a great way to relieve stress, boost your mood, and improve your overall well-being.

Incorporating movement into your daily routine is another effective strategy. This doesn't have to be a formal workout; simple actions like taking the stairs, walking during your lunch break, or doing a quick stretch session while watching TV all add up. These small bursts of activity can make a big difference over time, especially on days when you're not able to fit in a full workout.

Lastly, don't forget about recovery. As you maintain your exercise routine, it's important to allow your body time to rest and repair. This means scheduling regular rest days, incorporating stretching and mobility work, and ensuring you're getting enough sleep. Proper recovery helps prevent injury, keeps your energy levels up, and ensures that you're ready to give your best effort during your workouts.

Embracing the Long-Term Mindset

Maintaining your results isn't about staying on a strict diet forever or pushing yourself to the limit in every workout. It's about finding balance and making healthy choices that you can sustain for life. This means accepting that there will be ups and downs, but knowing that you have the tools to navigate them successfully.

The most important thing is to stay connected to your goals and to the reasons why you started this journey. Keep setting new challenges for yourself, whether it's trying a new recipe, increasing your weights at the gym, or simply drinking more water each day. Celebrate your successes, no matter how small, and remember that every positive choice you make is a step towards a healthier, happier you.

By staying adaptable, keeping your goals in focus, and continuing to prioritize your health, you can maintain your results and enjoy the benefits of your hard work for years to come.

2. BUILDING A SUPPORT SYSTEM

One of the most powerful tools in maintaining your weight loss and sustaining a healthy lifestyle is the support system you build around yourself. This isn't just about having people cheer you on—it's about creating a network that provides motivation, accountability, and guidance. A well-rounded support system can be the difference between short-term success and lifelong health. Whether it's through accountability partners, online communities, or professional guidance, the people you surround yourself with can help you stay on track, navigate challenges, and celebrate your victories.

Finding Accountability Partners

An accountability partner is someone who shares your commitment to health and fitness and helps keep you on track. This partnership is built on mutual support, encouragement, and a shared commitment to your goals. Finding the right person to share this journey with can make all the difference, turning what could be a solitary effort into a collaborative and motivating experience.

When looking for an accountability partner, consider someone whose goals align with yours. This could be a friend, family member, coworker, or even a neighbor. The key is to choose someone who is as committed as you are, someone who will not only encourage you but also hold you accountable when your motivation wanes. This relationship should be based on mutual respect, where both parties feel comfortable discussing successes and setbacks.

Regular check-ins are essential to the effectiveness of this partnership. Whether it's a daily text, a weekly phone call, or a monthly in-person meeting, consistent communication keeps you both engaged and accountable. During these check-ins, share your progress, discuss any challenges, and set goals for the upcoming period. This ongoing dialogue ensures that you stay focused and motivated, knowing that someone else is invested in your success.

It's also beneficial to engage in activities together. Working out as a team, attending a cooking class, or even prepping meals together can make the process more enjoyable and less daunting. The shared experience not only strengthens your bond but also reinforces your commitment to your health goals. Remember, the aim is to support each other through the highs and lows of your journey, celebrating victories and learning from setbacks together.

Joining Online Communities

In today's digital age, online communities offer a wealth of support, inspiration, and resources. These communities bring together people from all walks of life who share similar goals, challenges, and successes. Whether you're looking for advice, inspiration, or just a place to vent, online communities can be a valuable component of your support system. When choosing an online community, look for groups that align with your specific goals and values. There are countless forums, social media groups, and online platforms dedicated to health, fitness, and weight management. Some are more general, while others focus on specific diets, exercise routines, or health challenges. The best community for you is one where you feel welcomed, understood, and supported.

Engaging with an online community provides a sense of connection that can be incredibly motivating. You can share your experiences, ask for advice, and offer support to others. This exchange of ideas and experiences fosters a sense of belonging, reminding you that you're not alone on this journey. The collective wisdom of the group can also be a valuable resource, offering new perspectives, tips, and strategies that you might not have considered on your own.

It's important to be an active participant in these communities. The more you engage, the more you'll benefit. Share your successes, ask questions, and don't be afraid to contribute your own advice and experiences. The act of helping others can be just as motivating as receiving support. Plus, you'll build connections with others who can become an additional layer of accountability and encouragement.

However, it's also important to navigate these communities with discernment. Not all advice will be applicable to your situation, and not all community members will share your values or approach. Be mindful of what resonates with you, and don't hesitate to move on from a group that doesn't feel supportive or aligned with your goals. The internet is vast, and there's no shortage of spaces where you can find the encouragement and support you need.

Seeking Professional Guidance

While peer support is invaluable, there's also a place for professional guidance in your support system. Professionals bring expertise and experience that can help you refine your approach, overcome specific challenges, and achieve your goals more efficiently. Depending on your needs, this guidance could come from a nutritionist, personal trainer, therapist, or even a coach specializing in behavior change.

A nutritionist or dietitian can offer personalized advice on how to maintain your weight and optimize your diet for long-term health. They can help you navigate the complexities of nutrition, ensuring that your diet meets your nutritional needs while supporting your weight maintenance goals. This is particularly important if you have specific health conditions or dietary restrictions that require expert attention.

Personal trainers are another valuable resource, particularly if exercise is a key component of your maintenance plan. A trainer can help you develop a workout routine that's challenging, effective, and sustainable. They can also provide motivation, correct your form, and introduce new exercises to keep your routine fresh and engaging. The accountability of regular sessions with a trainer can also be a strong motivator to stay consistent with your exercise regimen.

Therapists or coaches who specialize in behavior change can help you address the mental and emotional aspects of weight maintenance. These professionals can offer strategies for managing stress, emotional eating, and other psychological barriers that might otherwise derail your progress. They can also help you set realistic goals, develop coping mechanisms, and build a mindset that supports long-term success.

When seeking professional guidance, it's important to choose someone who understands your goals and has the expertise to help you achieve them. Look for professionals with credentials, experience, and a communication style that resonates with you. The relationship should be one of collaboration and trust, where you feel comfortable discussing your challenges and confident in the advice you receive.

Regular check-ins with these professionals can keep you on track and help you make necessary adjustments as your needs evolve. They can offer fresh perspectives, troubleshoot issues, and provide the encouragement you need to stay committed to your health goals.

Whether it's a monthly session with a nutritionist, weekly workouts with a trainer, or regular therapy appointments, professional guidance can be the anchor that keeps you steady as you navigate the ups and downs of weight maintenance.

Building a support system is about surrounding yourself with the right people—those who will lift you up, keep you accountable, and guide you towards your goals. Whether through an accountability partner, an online community, or professional guidance, these connections can make your journey to long-term success not only achievable but also enjoyable. Remember, you don't have to do this alone. By tapping into the power of a strong support system, you set yourself up for sustained health and happiness.

3. ADAPTING TO LIFE CHANGES

Life is full of changes, and adapting to them is crucial for maintaining your health and fitness over the long term. Whether it's a new job, a move to a different city, changes in family dynamics, or even just the natural shifts that come with aging, your ability to adjust your plan to fit new circumstances can make all the difference. The key to long-term success lies in staying flexible, open-minded, and committed to embracing a healthy lifestyle for life.

Adjusting Your Plan for New Circumstances

Life rarely stays the same for long, and neither should your approach to health and fitness. As your circumstances change, your diet, exercise routine, and overall wellness strategy may need to shift to accommodate these new realities. The first step in adjusting your plan is recognizing when a change is necessary. This could be prompted by a significant life event, such as starting a new job with different hours, welcoming a new member to the family, or dealing with an injury or health condition.

When faced with these changes, take a moment to reassess your goals. What worked for you before may no longer be feasible, and that's okay. For example, if a new job requires you to work late hours, your previous evening workout routine might no longer be realistic. Instead, consider morning workouts or incorporating physical activity into your lunch break. Similarly, if you're dealing with a health issue, you might need to modify your diet or exercise plan to support your recovery while still maintaining your overall goals.

Adjusting your plan doesn't mean lowering your standards; it means being smart about how you approach your health in light of your new circumstances. For instance, if time becomes a constraint, focus on meal prepping on the weekends or choosing quick, healthy meals that can be thrown together in minutes. If your physical capabilities change, explore new forms of exercise that accommodate your current abilities while still challenging you. The goal is to find ways to stay consistent with your healthy habits, even when life throws you a curveball.

It's also essential to recognize the mental and emotional impact of life changes. Stress, anxiety, and even excitement can influence your behavior and motivation. During these times, give yourself grace. It's normal to experience setbacks, but the important thing is how you respond to them. Use these moments as an opportunity to recalibrate rather than abandon your efforts. Remember, adapting to life changes is about finding a new normal that works for you, not striving for perfection.

Staying Flexible and Open-Minded

Flexibility isn't just about physical ability; it's a mindset that allows you to navigate life's twists and turns with resilience and creativity. Staying flexible in your approach to health and wellness means being open to trying new things, letting go of rigid expectations, and embracing the idea that there are multiple paths to success.

One of the most important aspects of staying flexible is being willing to experiment with different strategies. What worked for you last year might not work this year, and that's okay. Maybe you were once an avid runner, but now your knees aren't up for the challenge.

Rather than giving up on exercise, explore alternatives like swimming, cycling, or yoga. Perhaps your dietary preferences or needs have changed—be open to experimenting with new foods, recipes, and meal plans that align with your current lifestyle.

Flexibility also involves being kind to yourself when things don't go as planned. Life is unpredictable, and there will be times when your best-laid plans fall apart. Rather than viewing these moments as failures, see them as opportunities to learn and grow. If you miss a workout or indulge in an unplanned treat, don't let it derail your progress. Instead, reflect on what happened, adjust your plan if necessary, and move forward with renewed determination.

Being open-minded also means staying informed and willing to adapt based on new information. The science of nutrition and fitness is always evolving, and what we know today may be different from what we knew a decade ago. Stay curious and willing to learn, whether it's about new exercise techniques, dietary trends, or wellness practices. However, also be discerning—filter out fads and focus on evidence-based strategies that align with your long-term goals.

Lastly, remember that flexibility doesn't mean a lack of commitment. It's about being adaptable while staying true to your overarching goal of living a healthy, balanced life. The more flexible and open-minded you are, the better equipped you'll be to navigate the inevitable changes life brings without losing sight of your wellness journey.

Embracing a Healthy Lifestyle for Life

The ultimate goal is to create a healthy lifestyle that you can sustain for the rest of your life. This isn't about following a strict diet or workout plan indefinitely, but rather about integrating healthy habits into your daily routine in a way that feels natural and enjoyable.

To embrace a healthy lifestyle for life, start by focusing on habits rather than outcomes. Instead of obsessing over the number on the scale or your performance in a particular workout, prioritize the daily actions that lead to long-term success. This could be as simple as making sure you get enough sleep, staying hydrated, eating a variety of nutrient-rich foods, and incorporating movement into your day. These small, consistent actions add up over time and become the foundation of a healthy life.

Another key to embracing a healthy lifestyle is to find joy in the process. Healthy living shouldn't feel like a chore—it should be something you look forward to. This means finding activities you love, foods you enjoy, and routines that fit naturally into your life. If you hate running, don't force yourself to run; try dancing, hiking, or playing a sport instead. If cooking feels like a burden, explore simple, delicious recipes that don't require hours in the kitchen. The more you enjoy the process, the more likely you are to stick with it long-term.

Social support is also critical to maintaining a healthy lifestyle. Surround yourself with people who encourage your healthy habits and share your values. This could be family, friends, or even an online community. Engage in activities together, share recipes, and celebrate each other's successes. Having a support system makes the journey more enjoyable and helps you stay accountable.

Finally, remember that a healthy lifestyle is about balance. There will be times when life gets busy, and your routine gets disrupted. That's okay. What matters is that you have the tools and mindset to get back on track when things settle down. Balance is about making healthy choices most of the time, but also allowing yourself the flexibility to enjoy life's pleasures without guilt.

In conclusion, adapting to life changes, staying flexible and open-minded, and embracing a healthy lifestyle for life are all interconnected. Each aspect supports the others, creating a robust framework that allows you to maintain your health and wellness regardless of what life throws your way. By focusing on these principles, you can ensure that your journey towards health is not just a phase, but a lifelong commitment that brings you joy, fulfillment, and well-being.

CONCLUSION

As we draw near the conclusion of our journey together in *The New Carb Cycling System*, it's essential to take a moment to reflect on the transformative steps we've taken. Embracing a lifestyle change as significant and promising as carb cycling is no minor feat, and you've done it with admirable commitment and perseverance.

Throughout this book, we have navigated the intricacies of carb cycling, unpacked the science, structured meal plans, and tackled both physical and emotional challenges. Each chapter was designed not only to provide you with the knowledge needed but to empower and equip you for a lifetime of healthier choices. The meal plans, the strategies to overcome cravings, and the incorporation of exercise are not just tools for weight loss, but for crafting a life brimming with energy and vitality.

Now, as you stand on this threshold, ready to carry forward the lessons and habits you've cultivated, remember that this is both an ending and a beginning. The conclusion of this book is not the conclusion of your journey. Instead, it's a gateway to further personal growth and exploration in your health and wellness path.

The steps you've taken will need to evolve as you do, adapting to life's inevitable changes and challenges. But the principles of carb cycling and the balanced approach you've learned provide a solid, flexible foundation that can adjust to these shifts. This adaptability underscores not just a diet change, but a lifestyle that caters to continual growth and adjustment, promoting long-term wellness.

As you move forward, hold on to the triumphs and lessons from your experiences. Let them remind you that while paths may bend and obstacles surface, your capacity to adapt and thrive remains unchanged. Remember, every meal, every choice is a stepping-stone to a healthier, more fulfilled you.

In the coming final pages, I'll share additional tips and resources to ensure you continue to feel supported and motivated as you write the subsequent chapters of your health story. Keep pushing forward, and remember, your journey is as unique and dynamic as you are.

REFLECTING ON YOUR JOURNEY

As you step back and survey the landscape of your personal health and wellness journey, it's crucial to acknowledge the significant strides and transformations you've undergone. Through the lens of carb cycling and structured meal planning, you've not only reshaped your eating habits but also, likely, your relationship with food and your body.

When you first opened this book, perhaps you were seeking a new path or a way to revitalize not just your diet, but your overall lifestyle. It's not just about fewer carbohydrates on some days or more on others; it's about understanding your body's needs and how it responds to different nutrients. This knowledge is powerful; it's transformative. It propels not merely a physical change but fosters a newfound respect and appreciation for the complexity and capability of your body.

Reflecting on your journey, think about the moments where you felt challenged. These could have been days when the low-carb plan felt particularly restricting, or when a high-carb day seemed counterintuitive to your weight loss goals. Each of these moments taught resilience and revealed the flexibility of the carb cycling system—a system that not only adjusts to your metabolic needs but also to your life's ebb and flow.

There's profound beauty in the awareness that your body is not a static entity; it is dynamic, responding daily to the energies and demands placed upon it. The past weeks have been your training ground, teaching you how to listen and adapt. Whether it was choosing the right kind of carbohydrate during a meal, understanding the importance of hydration, or balancing macros to fit your energy needs, each decision played a crucial role in advancing toward your goals.

Throughout these weeks, many of you have shared stories of heightened energy, better control over cravings, and a clearer understanding of how food can be both nourishing and enjoyable. This doesn't mean the path was free from obstacles. Days of frustration, moments of temptation, and the inevitable plateaus tested your resolve. Yet, here you are, having pushed through these barriers, perhaps more resilient and committed than ever.

This journey has also likely illuminated the importance of setting realistic, tangible goals. Carb cycling isn't just a method; it's a tool that works in sync with goal-setting. How you defined and measured success played a direct role in your motivation and perseverance. Remember, small, consistent wins pave the way to significant achievements. Celebrating these milestones, whether it involved fitting into an old pair of jeans, improving your cardiovascular health, or simply not feeling exhausted by mid-afternoon, each is a testament to your dedication.

Equally important in this journey has been your growing understanding of emotional eating and how to manage cravings effectively. The strategies discussed were designed not just to cope but to thrive; turning away from temporary comforts towards long-lasting rewards. Learning to distinguish between hunger and emotional needs is a critical step toward sustainable weight management and overall well-being.

Embracing mindful eating practices have, hopefully, turned your meals from mindless consumption into moments of genuine connection with your food. This mindfulness enriches the eating experience, augmenting not just the taste but also your body's response to food, enhancing metabolic flexibility and satisfaction levels.

As you reflect on these past chapters, remember each meal, each choice was part of a broader narrative—a narrative that you have authored through commitment, trial, and error, and continual learning. You've tailored the frameworks provided to fit your unique lifestyle, responsibilities, and needs, crafting a version of carb cycling that is distinctly yours.

In moving forward, use this reflection not just as a celebration of past successes but as a bulwark against future challenges. The tools, strategies, and insights you've gained are now an intrinsic part of your lifestyle toolkit. They will help you navigate future temptations and hurdles with greater ease and confidence.

Hold onto the lessons about nutritional balance, the importance of physical activity, and the psychological strategies that helped you manage stress and emotional eating. These are your allies as you continue to write your journey toward health and well-being.

And as we prepare to close this chapter, remember that every end is simply the beginning of another adventure. Armed with knowledge, experience, and a supportive community, you are more than equipped to continue this journey. Your path to health and wellness, like all great journeys, is ongoing—a beautiful, perpetual voyage that promises new lessons and uncharted terrains.

Embrace it with the enthusiasm and open-mindedness you showed when you first started carb cycling, and continue to nurture your body and mind with the care and respect they deserve. This isn't just a diet—it's a lifelong commitment to living well.

ENCOURAGEMENT FOR CONTINUED SUCCESS

Imagine standing at the threshold of your journey, looking back at the miles trekked and forward to the path yet to be explored. This visualization isn't just a reflection; it's an act of gearing up, fueled by achievements and learned lessons, ready to confront what lies ahead with a heartier, more seasoned approach. Your venture through *The New Carb Cycling System* has not just been about shedding weight or shaping up, but about instilling a resilience and adaptability that extends well beyond dietary choices.

The path to continued success with your carb cycling lifestyle is akin to tending a garden—a journey that requires patience, nurturing, and constant attention. It's about cultivating a vibrant lifestyle that continues to thrive season after season.

First, embrace the cyclical nature of your diet as a metaphor for life. Just as there are high and low carb days, life has its peaks and valleys. Success isn't found in avoiding these ups and downs but in navigating them with grace and adjusting your strategies as needed. Your ability to adapt your carb cycling to your changing body, emotions, and life circumstances will be crucial. Be as flexible and forgiving with yourself as you are rigorous in your planning.

Moreover, sustainable success is often rooted in community and connectivity. You're not just an individual on a diet but a member of a collective journey of wellness. Reach out and share your experiences. Engaging in forums, local groups, or online communities can offer support, deepen your understanding, and, importantly, affirm that you're not alone in your struggles or victories.

A pivotal element to sustaining your enthusiasm and drive is setting new goals. Just as you've met and possibly exceeded your initial targets, continuing to challenge yourself is imperative. These goals don't always need to be monumental. Small, achievable goals can provide ongoing motivation and satisfaction, ensuring that every small win fuels your drive to maintain this lifestyle.

Reflect on the educational aspect of your journey—the nutritional insights, the understanding of metabolic responses, and the holistic view of how lifestyle influences your well-being. Continue to educate yourself. The landscapes of health, nutrition, and fitness are ever-expanding, with new studies, technologies, and methodologies continually emerging. Staying informed empowers you to make adjustments that align with the latest research, enhancing both your results and your journey.

Another vital aspect of sustained success involves anticipation and preemptive strategy. Anticipate potential setbacks like holidays, emotional upheavals, or busy periods at work.

Having a proactive approach, whether it's adjusting your meal plans in advance or ramping up your support systems during these times, can make all the difference. Such preparedness prevents backsliding and keeps you moving forward, even through challenging periods.

Mindfulness, a cornerstone of your initial success, continues to play an integral role. Being mindful about each meal and snack isn't just about staying within a carb limit; it's about deepening your connection with your body's signals and needs. Eat slowly, savor each bite, and listen—really listen—to how food affects your mood, energy levels, and physical health. This ongoing conversation between you and your body is foundational in fine-tuning your diet to best serve you.

Furthermore, revisit your relationship with exercise. Integrating physical activity that you enjoy can significantly enhance your carb cycling results and general well-being. Whether it's finding new sports, joining classes, or even taking up mindful yoga, make physical activity a joyful and expected part of your daily routine.

Finally, embrace the imperfections along the way. No journey is void of missteps, and each one offers valuable lessons. Learn from them without self-rebuke. Growth is not in flawless execution but in persistent effort, resilience, and the wisdom to adapt from experiences—one meal, one day at a time.

Remember, this book isn't just a manual you read once but a companion to refer back to as you forge ahead. Your journey with carb cycling is as dynamic and evolving as you are. Every day presents a new opportunity to reinforce your commitment, refine your approach, and recommit to your wellness goals. With every choice, you continue to author your story—a story of health, resilience, and continual transformation.

Thus, carry forward with confidence, nurtured by the habits and insights you've gained. You are equipped, empowered, and, above all, accompanied by hundreds finding their way alongside you. Here's to a continuum of success, health, and discovery—beyond just weight loss, into a lifetime of thriving and optimal well-being.

FINAL TIPS AND RESOURCES

As you step beyond the structured confines of this book, weaving the principles of carb cycling into the fabric of your daily life, a few final tips and resources can serve as guideposts to assist you in maintaining your newfound lifestyle. These encapsulate not just advice on continuing your dietary approach but encompass a broader spectrum of tools designed to support, inspire, and cultivate your journey towards lasting wellness.

Embarking on this path, you've learned that knowledge is not just power—it's empowerment. Continuing to educate yourself on the nuances of nutrition and the ever-evolving insights into human health will equip you with the ability to make informed decisions that benefit your body and mind. Subscribe to journals, listen to podcasts, and follow influencers in the health and fitness realms who base their advice on scientifically validated research. This ongoing education will serve as your radar, helping you navigate through vast seas of information, discerning fact from fad.

Toolkits vary from one individuaL to another, and an integral component of yours may involve digital tools. Technology can simplify the complex, making what seems daunting decidedly manageable.

Apps for tracking meals and nutrients, for instance, can help you monitor your carb cycling with precision, removing guesswork and ensuring consistency. Other apps that log physical activity or provide virtual workout sessions can also align neatly with your goals, offering convenience and customization.

In addition to digital tools, consider maintaining a physical or an electronic journal. Documenting your journey provides more than just a record; it offers insights into what works, what doesn't, and how your body and emotions respond to various changes. Over time, this journal becomes a treasure trove of personalized data, guiding your decisions and adjustments.

Support systems are not merely adjuncts to your journey—they can be central to your success. If possible, engage a nutritionist who understands carb cycling or a personal trainer who respects the nutritional side of your fitness regime. For many, however, professional advice isn't always accessible or affordable. In such cases, online communities about carb cycling, healthy eating, and lifestyle changes can be invaluable. These platforms allow you to share experiences, gain moral and informational support, and learn from others who are at various stages of their own journeys.

Your physical environment is also part of your toolkit. Creating a home environment that supports your health goals—be it through stocking healthy foods, setting up a small home gym, or simply having a dedicated space for meditation and relaxation—can significantly influence your daily choices. When your environment echoes your health aspirations, staying on track becomes a tad easier.

Another substantial resource is your local library or bookstore. Here, you can find books not only about diets and nutrition but also about behavioral change, stress management, and the science of habit formation. Understanding these broader topics can enhance your ability to stick with carb cycling and manage the psychological challenges that come with lifestyle changes.

The role of mental health in physical health cannot be overstressed. Engaging in regular mindfulness practices, be it through guided meditations, yoga, or deep breathing exercises, can enhance your emotional resilience and capacity to maintain lifestyle changes. Remember, stress can sabotage even the most nutritionally sound diet, so integrating stress management techniques is crucial.

Lastly, as your journey evolves, so might your dietary needs and preferences. Stay open to tweaking your carb cycling plan. You might find that certain adjustments—maybe shifting the ratio of your macronutrients, altering your high-carb days, or even the timing of your meals—better support your health as it improves or as your lifestyle changes.

To encapsulate, moving forward with confidence in the carb cycling lifestyle means more than just remembering the specifics of meal planning. It involves a holistic approach to wellness that integrates continuous learning, supportive tools and communities, conducive environments, and robust strategies for both physical and mental health.

Carry these resources and tips with you as a compass and map, guiding your path and helping you navigate your health journey, one thoughtful choice at a time. Here's to not just achieving but living your success, basking in the vitality and vibrance of well-being that you've worked so ardently to cultivate. Remember, this is not the end but a bright continuation of a fulfilling quest toward your best health.

Made in the USA
Las Vegas, NV
25 January 2025

16954266R10059